U0218988

EMERGENCY HOSPITALS FOR COVID-19

CONSTRUCTION AND OPERATION MANUAL

新冠应急医院

建设运营手册

阎　志　主编

Yan Zhi　　Editor-in-Chief

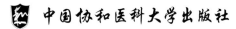
中国协和医科大学出版社

图书在版编目（CIP）数据

新冠应急医院建设运营手册 / 阎志主编. —北京：中国协和医科大学出版社，2020.6

ISBN 978-7-5679-1538-1

Ⅰ.①新… Ⅱ.①阎… Ⅲ.①传染病医院-建筑设计-手册 Ⅳ.①TU246.1-62

中国版本图书馆CIP数据核字（2020）第083320号

新冠应急医院建设运营手册

主　　编：阎　志
责任编辑：顾良军

出版发行　**中国协和医科大学出版社**
　　　　　（北京市东城区东单三条9号　邮编100730　电话010-65260431）
网　　址：www.pumcp.com
经　　销：新华书店总店北京发行所
印　　刷：中煤（北京）印务有限公司

开　　本：889×1194　1/32
印　　张：5.625
字　　数：130千字
版　　次：2020年6月第1版
印　　次：2020年6月第1次印刷
定　　价：80.00元

ISBN 978-7-5679-1538-1

总　目　录

EMERGENCY HOSPITALS

HOSPITALS

FOR COVID-19

CONSTRUCTION AND
OPERATION MANUAL

新冠应急医院
建 设 运 营 手 册

阎 志 主编

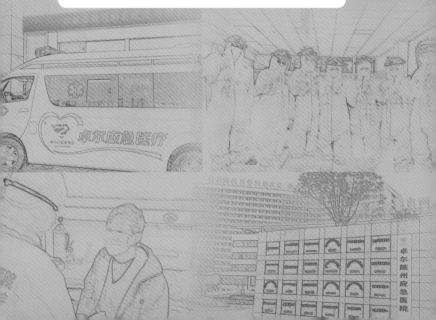

主　　编：阎　志

编写人员：阎　志　张　亮　杜书伟　田旭东

　　　　　牛亚冬　熊小川

英文翻译：阎　格

英文审校：王斯达

版式设计：黄　萱　宋　杰　叶芹云　胡杨苻

摄　　影：范睿奇

前　言

新型冠状病毒（SARS-CoV-2）是一种新出现的病原体，具有传染性强、传播速度快的特点，在无防护下通过飞沫和密切接触在感染者和被感染者之间发生传播。中国和世界其他国家及地区均出现了新型冠状病毒肺炎（COVID-19）疫情。

面对新冠肺炎疫情的暴发，在专业传染病医院收治能力严重不足的情况下，卓尔公益基金会提出建设新冠应急医院，将不具备传染病患者收治能力或收治能力不足的医院迅速改造为可用于集中收治疑似和确诊新型冠状病毒肺炎患者的应急医院。新冠应急医院的出现，有效缓解了当地传染病医院床位不足、收治不足的问题，在疫情防治中发挥了一定的作用。

本手册由卓尔公益基金会组织参与新冠应急医院改造、保障服务相关人员，对新冠应急医院的建设运营经验进行整理归纳，并参考相关医疗管理规范、标准编写而成，以期为全球各地区在紧急改造现有医疗机构，扩增医疗资源方面提供借鉴，助力有效应对新冠疫情。

阎　志

卓尔公益基金会创始人

2020年4月

目　　录

第一章 新冠应急医院建设背景

1.1 新冠应急医院的产生

传染病是一类由各类病原体引起的，可以借助一定途径在人与人之间进行传播的疾病，其中呼吸道传染病的传染性最强，对人群健康危害最大。

传染病的治疗对医疗环境和防护措施有较高的要求，需要在特定的传染病医院完成，以防普通疾病患者和医护人员被感染。传染病的发生率相对较低，随着医学技术的发展和公共卫生治理的完善，传染病的暴发和扩散得到了有效抑制，因而常态下传染病医院在数量和规模上要远远小于普通医院；但也正因如此，传染病一旦发生大流行，相应的医疗资源往往不足。2020年初，新型冠状病毒肺炎在短时间内发生了大规模的传播，使得世界范围内的传染病医疗资源出现了严重短缺的问题。

新型冠状病毒肺炎疫情暴发后，湖北省武汉市定点传染病医院爆满，已有的医疗资源不能满足新增患者的救治需求。在此情况下，卓尔公益基金会提出联合专业医疗机构，共同设立"新冠应急医院"的方案，并迅速与不具备传染病患者收治能力或收治能力不足的武汉市第八医院、武汉市汉阳医院、黄冈市中心医院大别山区域医疗中心、黄陂区人民医院盘龙城分院、罗田县第二人民医院、监利县人民医院和随州市中心医院等7家医院开展合作，在最短时间内将其改造为收治新冠肺炎患者的应急医院。卓尔7家新冠应急医院的改造中，最短的医院改造仅用了2天时间，最长的也只用了5天时间。改造完成后共开放床位4583个，累计治愈武汉、黄冈、随州、荆州等地新冠肺炎确诊及疑似患者2833例。

新冠应急医院因新冠肺炎疫情而建成，仅集中收治新冠肺炎确诊及疑似患者。这种将已有医疗机构迅速改造为专业收治新冠肺炎患者的应急医院模式，缓解了疫区医疗资源紧缺的问题，提高了疫区医院的收治能力，有效弥补了防疫工作的短板，在患者救治和医疗保障中发挥了重要作用。

1.2 新冠应急医院的定义

新冠应急医院是为有效应对新冠肺炎疫情，将不具备传染病收治能力或收治能力不足的综合医院进行改造后，用于专门收治新冠肺炎患者的应急医院，在环境布局、设备设施和管理制度等方面与专业传染病医院具有相等水平。新冠应急医院的主要目标是解决新冠肺炎确诊及疑似患者不能得到有效隔离治疗的问题，从而控制传染源，防止疾病发生更大范围的流行。新冠应急医院是由现有医疗机构改造而成，具有快速建设、成本较低的特点，可以迅速解决疫区传染病医疗资源不足的问题。

1.3 新冠应急医院的功能

（1）新冠肺炎患者筛查和分诊

新冠应急医院通过开设发热门诊，对发热患者进行实验室检查、影像学检查和流行病学调查，从而准确区分普通发热患者、新冠肺炎疑似患者和新冠肺炎确诊患者，并根据患者病情进行分诊和收治。

（2）新冠肺炎疑似患者隔离观察和治疗

通过发热门诊筛查出的新冠肺炎疑似患者，在通过核酸检测确诊之前，由新冠应急医院进行单独隔离观察和治疗，以防其感染普通人群或被新冠肺炎确诊患者感染。

（3）新冠肺炎确诊患者收治和转运

新冠应急医院对自身筛查出的新冠肺炎患者或由其他医疗机构转运来的新冠肺炎患者进行隔离收治，直至患者达到出院标准。对于病情发生恶化、而新冠应急医院自身不具备救治能力的患者，则将其快速转运至更高级别的新冠肺炎定点医院进行救治。

第二章 新冠应急医院工程设计

新冠应急医院的设计应符合现行有关标准的规定。本部分内容主要以《传染病医院建筑设计规范》（GB 50849-2014）《传染病医院建设标准》（建标173-2016）等规范、要求为基础进行设计。

2.1 医院环境设计

（1）新冠应急医院应设置具有引导、管理等功能的标识系统。

（2）新冠应急医院应满足无障碍通行的需求。

（3）医院布局应严格划分限制区域与隔离区域，区域之间应采取物理分隔并设置道闸。限制区域主要规划生活用房及后勤保障用房，隔离区域主要规划接诊用房、医技用房、住院用房及空气吸引、医用垃圾焚烧装置、临时停尸房及污水处理站等配套用房。限制区域应位于隔离区域的上风向。

（4）所有建筑平面布局应严格按照"三区两通道"划分。"三区"即污染区、半污染区（又称"潜在污染区"）和清洁区。清洁区是不易受到患者血液、体液和病原微生物等物质污染及传染病患者不应进入的区域；半污染区位于清洁区与污染区之间，是有可能被患者血液、体液和病原微生物等物质污染的区域；污染区是传染病患者和疑似传染病患者接受诊疗的区域，包括被其血液、体液、分泌物、排泄物污染物品暂存和处理的场所。必须明确医务人员内部作业流线：按清洁区→半污染区→污染区单向作业流程布置，相邻区域之间应设置相应的卫生通过或缓冲室并配备洗手盆和污衣桶，以确保医务人员不被感染。"两通道"即医务人员通道和患者通道，清洁物流和污染物流分设专用路线，避免交叉。医务人员通道及出入口应设在清洁区一端，患者通道及出入口应设在污染区一端。

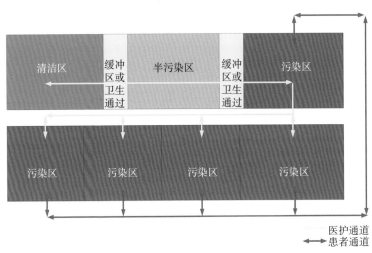

图2-1　"三区两通道"设计

（5）医疗主体建筑的布局应考虑接诊、医技、住院等主要部门间的功能联系安全便捷、合理高效。

（6）建筑间距应满足感染控制和卫生隔离的要求，隔离区域与限制区域相互间距宜大于30米，隔离区域内建筑间距宜大于20米。

（7）应根据医院规模设置至少2个出入口，主要出入口应避免布置在交通主要干道上，院区救护车出入口附近应设置救护车洗消场地和设施。

（8）污水处理站应布置在院区地势较低，且便于把经严格消毒处理达标后的污水排向城市排水管网的位置。

2.2 接诊区设计

（1）应靠近院区的主要出入口。

（2）门诊入口处应明显划分筛查区域，以避免就诊空间过分拥挤而致使就诊患者之间产生交叉感染。

（3）医务人员进出接诊工作区的出入口部应设置卫生通过。

（4）应设置诊室、留观室、X线室、B超室、心电室、治疗（配制）室、污物暂存间、消毒间、洁具间、医务人员值班室、更衣室、医生办公室、医生卫生间等。

（5）除诊室、X线室、B超室、心电室可同时向医护通道、患者通道开门外，其他医用房间仅可向医护通道开门。

（6）宜设置从门诊直接通往住院入口的患者通道，避免其再次经过其他区域感染他人。

2.3 病区设计

（1）有条件的宜设置一定数量的负压隔离病房和重症监护病房（ICU）隔离负压小间，用于收治复杂病情患者、危重症患者或具有超级传播特性的患者。

（2）有条件的宜设置多学科联合会诊室和远程医疗会诊室。

（3）应根据患者的感染程度（疑似患者、轻症患者和重症患者）分设不同病区和病房：疑似病区应采用单人病房；确诊病区可采用单人或多人病房；复杂病情患者、危重症患者或具有超级传播特性的患者应采用单人负压隔离病房。

（4）每个病区的工作区内应设护士站、治疗室、处置室、医生办公室、护士办公室、值班室、消毒间、污洗间、被服库房、病人备餐间、开水间等。

2.4　病房设计

（1）病床的排列应平行于有采光窗的墙面，单间一般布置1～2床，有条件的尽量调整为单床间。

（2）多床病房中，平行的两床间净距不应小于1.10m，靠墙病床床沿与墙面的净距不应小于0.80m。

（3）单排病床通道净宽不应小于1.10m。

（4）各病房均应附设含大便器、淋浴器、脸盆的卫生间。

（5）病房门应直接开向走道。

（6）抢救室宜靠近护士站。

（7）病房门净宽不应小于1.10m，门扇应设观察窗。

（8）病房应保持最佳通风状态，最基本的要求是窗户直接通向外界，方便开窗通风；或设有通风、送风设备。

（9）病房走道两侧墙面应设置靠墙扶手及防撞设施。

（10）病房与医护通道之间应设置观察窗和传递窗，传递窗宜采用双门密闭联动传递窗。

2.5　医技科室设计

（1）平面布置应区分病人等候检查区与医务人员诊断工作区，并应在医务人员进出诊断工作区设置卫生通过。

（2）集中药库、药房应设置在清洁区，护理单元药品间可设置在半污染区。

2.6　电气和智能化设计

（1）负压隔离病房区的电源应按区域单独供电，负压隔离病房的强弱电电气设备的所有管路、接线盒应采用可靠的密封措施，负压隔离病房照明控制应采用就地与清洁区两地控制。

（2）病区应按清洁区、半污染区、污染区分别设置配电回路，主要电气装置应布置在清洁区内。

（3）负压隔离病房和洁净用房的照明灯具应采用洁净密闭型灯具，并宜吸顶安装；当嵌入安装时，其安装缝隙应采取可靠的密封措施。灯罩应采用不易破损、透光好的材料。照明灯具应表面光洁，易于消毒。

（4）清洁走廊、污洗间、卫生间、候诊室、诊室、治疗室、病房、手术室及其他需要灭菌消毒的地方应设紫外线消毒器或杀菌灯。紫外线杀菌灯应有防误开措施，其开关安装高度底部距地 1.80m。

2.7　给水和排水设计

（1）污染区、半污染区与清洁区的排水管和通气管应独立设置，排水管道应采用防腐蚀的管道。

（2）给水、热水的配水干管、支管设置的检修阀门，宜设在工作人员的清洁区和半污染区内，严禁设置在污染区内。

（3）所有卫生器具、地漏均应设置水封，且不得小于50mm，应封闭不常用地漏。

（4）传染病区的雨水宜收集至雨水蓄水池，消毒合格后再排放至城市雨水管网。

（5）病区的污废水应统一收集，经预消毒后排入化粪池，再进入医院污水处理站。污水站应采用二级生化处理工艺，出水消毒合格后再排入城市污水管网。

2.8 采暖通风与空气调节设计

（1）应设置机械通风系统，且应为管道通风。为避免交叉感染，机械送、排风系统应按清洁区、半污染区、污染区分区独立设置。

（2）负压隔离病房最小换气次数应为12次/小时，污染区、半污染区最小换气次数应为6次/小时，清洁区最小换气次数应为3次/小时。

（3）空调冷凝水应集中收集，并应排入消毒池，消毒处理后排入医院污水处理站。

（4）如使用空调，每间隔离病房空调末端应能独立运行。如果同一空调末端负担多个病房，应立即停止使用，并对该类病房加装分体式空调机或VRF多联机。

（5）机械送、排风系统应使病区内空气压力从清洁区至半污染区至污染区依次降低。隔离病房与其相邻、相通的缓冲室、走廊压差，应保持不小于5Pa的负压差。每间隔离病房要在清洁区的缓冲室墙上加装微压测压计。

（6）清洁区、半污染区气流组织可为上送上排方式。隔离病房内应改建为上送下排方式：送风口建议设于床尾处顶送，排风口设于床头处下排。

（7）负压隔离病房的送排风系统宜独立设置，送排风系统的过滤器设置压差检测、报警装置。当集中设置时，每个系统服务的病房数量不宜超过6间。

（8）病房的送风应经过粗效、中效、亚高效三级处理后送入室内。排风应经过高效过滤器处理后排放，排风高效过滤器应设置于病房排风口处。

（9）隔离病房的排风出口改造宜高于屋面3m以上，应远离任何进风口和门窗20m以上，并处于其下风向；通风系统排风机位置的设置必须保证建筑物内排风管道保持负压；负压隔离病房通风系统的送、排风机应连锁控制，启动通风系统时应先启动排风机再启动送风机，关闭通风系统时应先关闭送风机再关闭排风机。

第三章　新冠应急医院工程改造

3.1　新冠应急医院改造流程

将普通医院改造为新冠应急医院主要经历以下几个步骤。见图3-1。

（1）转移非新冠肺炎患者

为避免医院现有非新冠肺炎住院患者受到感染，在改造前应将该部分患者转移至其他普通医院或送至家中治疗休养。

（2）评估医院现况，分析改造内容

从医院环境、病区布局、病房设计、供水排水等几个方面对医院的现况进行评估，并结合新冠应急医院建设标准，分析需要进一步改造的内容。

（3）设计施工方案

结合上述评估和分析结果，设计医院改造的施工方案。

（4）施工改造

以施工方案为基础，筹备物料和设备，并对医院各个方面进行逐一改造。

（5）交付运营

施工改造完成后，对改造结果进行评估验收，如验收合格，则可交付运营，开展新冠肺炎患者的收治工作。

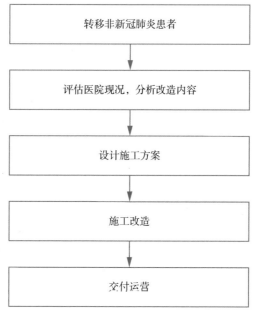

图3-1　新冠应急医院改造流程

3.2　新冠应急医院改造方案

将已有医院及设施进行临时、局部、快速改造为能够收治新冠肺炎患者的应急医院，是扩增新冠肺炎医疗资源，提高新冠肺炎隔离、治疗能力的重要手段。新冠应急医院的改造方案应严格参照新冠应急医院布局设计来制定。

3.2.1　医院环境改造

（1）医院严格划分污染区、半污染区和清洁区。明确医务人员内部作业流线，在相邻区域之间设置相应的卫生通过或缓冲室并配备洗手盆和污衣桶。

（2）严格规划和区分医务人员通道和患者通道，分别设置清洁物流专用路线和污染物流专用路线。医务人员通道及出入口设在清洁区一端，患者通道及出入口设在污染区一端。

（3）在原有医院的基础上设置传染病防控专用通道，并设隔离设施。

（4）清理新冠应急医院建筑或建筑周边与疫情防控无关的设施和停车，对于安全距离不满足规范要求（小于20m）的附近建筑，采取必要的隔离措施或暂停使用，明显位置标识隔离区。

（5）划分并标识防疫物品装卸场地和临时堆放场地。

（6）划分并标识救护车的清洗和消毒场地。

（7）对医疗废弃物及污废水处理站，采取进一步的环境安全保护措施。

3.2.2 接诊区改造

（1）在医院入口处设置发热门诊。

（2）按照"三区两通道"原则对接诊区进行布局。

（3）在门诊入口处划分出筛查区域。

（4）确保接诊区具备诊室、留观室、X线室、B超室、心电室、治疗（配制）室、污物暂存间、消毒间、洁具间、医务人员值班室、更衣室、医生办公室、医生卫生间等。

（5）除诊室、X线室、B超室、心电室外，将其他医用房间设置为仅可向医护通道开门。

（6）设置从门诊直接通往住院入口的患者通道。

3.2.3 病区改造

（1）按照"三区两通道"原则对病区进行布局改造。

（2）有条件的宜增设一定数量的负压隔离病房和重症监护病房（ICU）隔离负压小间。

（3）有条件的宜增设多学科联合会诊室和远程医疗会诊室。

（4）分设不同病区和病房用于安置不同感染程度的患者。

（5）确保每个病区的工作区内设有护士站、治疗室、处置室、医生办公室、护士办公室、值班室、消毒间、污洗间、被服库房、病人备餐间、开水间等。

3.2.4　普通隔离病房改造

（1）多床病房中，平行的两床间净距不小于1.10m，靠墙病床床沿与墙面的净距不小于0.80m。

（2）单排病床通道净宽不小于1.10m。

（3）确保病房内设置氧气、吸引等床头治疗设施及呼叫、对讲设施，确保床边有足够空间放置床边X线机、呼吸机等设备。

（4）病房与医护通道之间设置观察窗和传递窗，传递窗宜采用双门密闭联动传递窗。

3.2.5　负压隔离病房改造

普通病房改造为负压隔离病房的方案如下（图3-2）。

（1）负压病房每间设置独立的卫生间，在医护走廊与病房之间设置缓冲前室，设置非手动或自动感应龙头洗手池，墙上设置双门密闭式传递窗。

（2）房间气流组织应当防止送、排风短路，送风口位置应当使清洁空气首先流过房间中医务人员可能的工作区域，然后流过传染源进入排风口。送风口应当设置在房间上部。病房、诊室等污染区的排风口设置在房间下部，房间排风口底部距地面不应小于100mm。

（3）每间负压隔离病房设置一套1500立方米/小时风量全新风系统。送风应经过粗效、中效、亚高效过滤器三级处理，且设两套排风系统，其中一套带高效过滤器。排风应当经过高效过滤器过滤处理后排放。排风的高效空气过滤器应当安装在房间排风口处。每间负压隔离病房的送、排风管上应当设置密闭阀。设传感系统控制变频风机，保证负压病房与缓冲、走廊保持5Pa负压。

（4）负压隔离病房为一级特别重要负荷。由现状变电所（配电室，电气竖井）不同的低压母线引两路电源为病房供电，其中一路引自应急段，在病房合适位置设一双电源配电箱为病房负荷供电；由本楼变电所（配电室，电气竖井）不同的低压母线引两路电源为病房通风系统供电，其中一路引自应急段，在病房通风系统合适位置设一双电源配电箱为病房通风系统供电。

（5）确保负压隔离病房通风系统的送、排风机为连锁控制。

（6）弱电智能化：

1）病房内原有的弱电系统（数据端口、电视端口、医护对讲、火灾探测器等）维持不变。

2）病房新增建筑设备监控系统，对通风系统进行自动控制，并应监视污染区及半污染区的压差。

3）病房新增门禁控制系统，对负压病房的医、患通道，污染与洁净区的过渡进行控制。

4）病房新增视频监护系统，采用语音及视频双向通信功能。

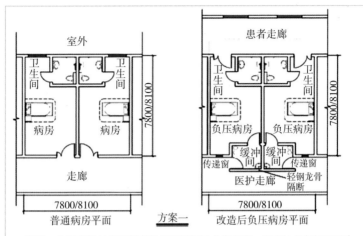

说明：负压病房与走廊间应设有双门密闭式传递窗，病室与走廊间设缓冲过渡小间，将门错开布置避免气流倒灌，缓冲间应设免洗消毒液，供医务人员进出病室消毒用，并设污物桶收集一次性废弃物。

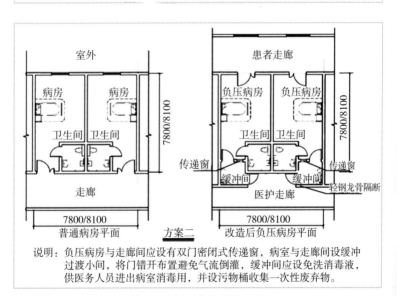

说明：负压病房与走廊间应设有双门密闭式传递窗，病室与走廊间设缓冲过渡小间，将门错开布置避免气流倒灌，缓冲间应设免洗消毒液，供医务人员进出病室消毒用，并设污物桶收集一次性废弃物。

图3-2　负压病房改造方案

3.2.6　医技科室改造

按照"三区两通道"原则对医技科室进行布局改造，将集中药库、药房设置在清洁区，护理单元药品间可设置在半污染区。明确区分病人等候检查区与医务人员诊断工作区，并在医务人员进出诊断工作区设置卫生通过。

3.2.7　电气和智能化改造

（1）病区按清洁区、半污染区、污染区分别设置配电回路，主要电气装置布置在清洁区内。

（2）负压隔离病房和洁净用房的照明灯具采用洁净密闭型灯具，并宜吸顶安装。

（3）在清洁走廊、污洗间、卫生间、候诊室、诊室、治疗室、病房、手术室及其他需要灭菌消毒的地方设置紫外线消毒器或杀菌灯。

3.2.8　给水和排水改造

（1）确保污染区、半污染区与清洁区的排水管和通气管为独立设置。

（2）将给水、热水的配水干管、支管设置的检修阀门，设在工作人员的清洁区和半污染区内。

（3）确保所有卫生器具、地漏均设有水封，且不得小于50mm，封闭不常用地漏。

（4）封闭诊室、护士室、治疗室、检查室、与病房隔离的洗手间等地的地漏。病房内卫生间可有地漏，但需定期检查，给地漏水封补水。

（5）确保室外污废水排水检查井采用密闭井盖。排水管网配设通气立管，通气口高出地面2.00m。

3.2.9 采暖通风与空气调节改造

（1）设置机械通风系统，且为管道通风。机械送、排风系统按清洁区、半污染区、污染区分区独立设置。

（2）负压隔离病房最小换气次数应为12次／小时，污染区、半污染区最小换气次数应为6次／小时，清洁区最小换气次数应为3次／小时。

（3）设置空调冷凝水集中收集装置，并与消毒池连接。

（4）确保每间隔离病房空调末端能独立运行。停止使用同时负担多个病房的空调，并对该类病房加装分体式空调机或VRF多联机。

（5）确保隔离病房与其相邻、相通的缓冲室、走廊保持不小于5Pa的负压差。在每间隔离病房清洁区的缓冲室墙上加装微压测压计。

（6）将隔离病房内改建为上送下排方式。

（7）确保病房的送风应经过粗效、中效、亚高效三级处理后送入室内，并设置排风高效过滤器于病房排风口处。

（8）将隔离病房的排风出口改造为高于屋面3m以上，远离任何进风口和门窗20m以上，并处于其下风向；通风系统排风机位置的设置必须保证建筑物内排风管道保持负压。

（9）确保病房区的污废水排水通气管未连接非病区的排水通气管。上屋面的通气管口处周边应当有良好的通风条件，有条件的在通气管口处配设气体消毒设施。

3.3 收治确诊患者的新冠应急医院改造案例

对于因疫情较重，医疗资源相对不足而导致确诊患者不能完全收治的地区，改造后的新冠应急医院主要用于收治确诊患者。本部分以卓尔长江应急医院（武汉市第八医院）、卓尔汉江应急医院（武汉市汉阳医院）为例，对收治确诊患者新冠应急医院的改造进行介绍。

3.3.1　卓尔长江应急医院

为缓解疫情暴发后医疗资源严重不足的局面，卓尔公益基金会与武汉市第八医院展开合作，对该医院北院进行紧急改造。2020 年 1 月 30 日，卓尔长江应急医院正式挂牌成立，这是第一家卓尔新冠应急医院。医院总计设置床位 300 张，主要用于收治新冠肺炎确诊患者，运营期间累计收治 560 人。医院改造的平面布局见图 3-3、图 3-4。

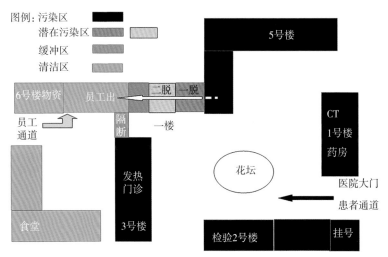

图3-3　卓尔长江应急医院一楼平面布局图

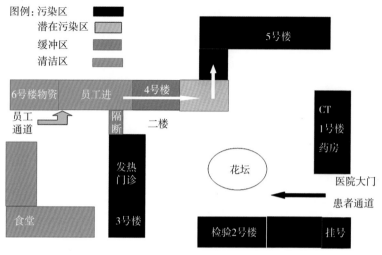

图3-4　卓尔长江应急医院二楼平面布局图

3.3.2　卓尔汉江应急医院

2020年2月1日，卓尔公益基金会与武汉市汉阳医院开展合作，设立卓尔汉江应急医院，主要用于收治新冠肺炎确诊患者。经过3天改造施工，将普通住院区按照规范标准改造为"三区两通道"的隔离病区。改造后的卓尔汉江应急医院新增床位260张，运营期间累计收治487人。医院的改造施工见图3-5、图3-6、图3-7。

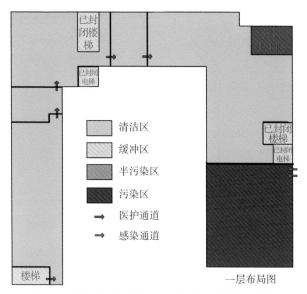

图3-5　卓尔汉江应急医院内科楼一层施工改造图

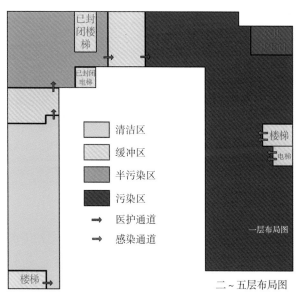

图3-6　卓尔汉江应急医院内科楼二~五层施工改造图

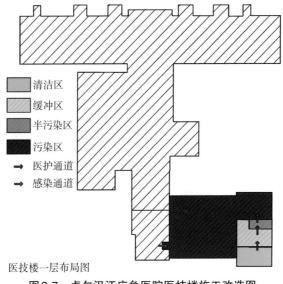

医技楼一层布局图

图3-7　卓尔汉江应急医院医技楼施工改造图

3.4　收治疑似患者的新冠应急医院改造案例

对于疫情相对较轻，医疗资源相对充足，确诊患者可以得到完全收治，而疑似患者不能完全收治的地区，为了实现分级治疗，有部分改造后的新冠应急医院主要用于收治疑似患者。本部分以卓尔盘龙城应急医院（黄陂区人民医院盘龙城分院）、卓尔罗田应急医院（罗田县第二人民医院）为例，对收治疑似患者新冠应急医院的改造进行介绍。

3.4.1　卓尔盘龙城应急医院

2020年2月7日，卓尔公益基金会与黄陂区人民医院联合设立卓尔盘龙城应急医院，将黄陂区人民医院盘龙城分院内科、儿科住院病房按照规范标准改造为"三区两通道"的隔离病区，共设100张床位，主要用于收治新冠肺炎疑似患者。运营期间累计收治358人，治愈123人。医院改造平面布局见图3-8。

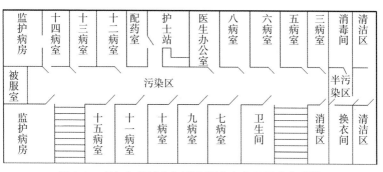

图3-8 卓尔盘龙城应急医院隔离病房平面分布设计

3.4.2 卓尔罗田应急医院

2020年2月7日，卓尔公益基金会与罗田县第二人民医院联合成立卓尔罗田应急医院。医院设有100间隔离病房，共计500张床位，主要用于收治新冠肺炎疑似患者，运营期间累计收治192人，治愈180人。医院改造平面布局见图3-9、图3-10。

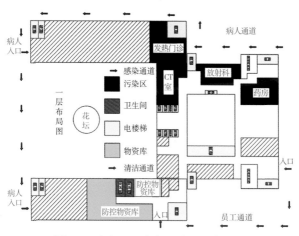

图3-9 卓尔罗田应急医院一层布局图

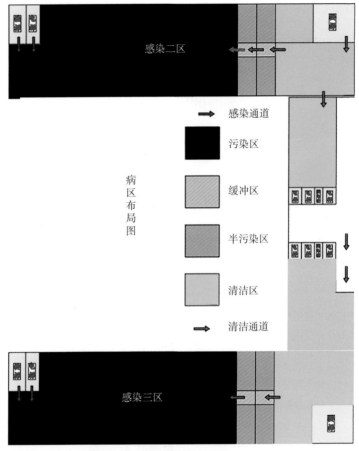

图3-10 卓尔罗田应急医院病区布局图

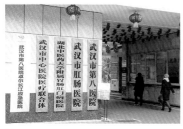

卓尔先后成立7家应急医院

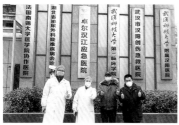
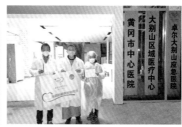

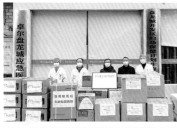
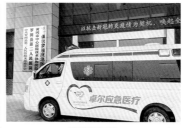

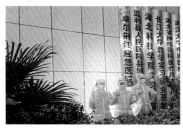
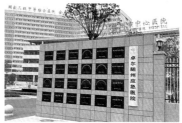

图3-11　卓尔应急医院

第四章　新冠应急医院运营

4.1　医务人员培训

4.1.1　编制规范化培训课程

医院组织临床科室中具有丰富抗击疫情和教学经验的骨干医生，以相关规范为基础，结合医院实际情况，严格制定培训课程和考核试题，主要内容包括正确手卫生，戴脱防护口罩、手套和防护目镜、面屏，穿脱防护服和隔离衣，分级防护、预检分诊台工作以及诊疗护理规范等操作流程。

4.1.2　培养同质化师资队伍

首先从医院临床技能训练中心的导师团队中遴选医生和护士作为培训师，并分三阶段进行培训，每个阶段实行组长负责制，由组长对所有培训师进行考核评估，确保师资队伍的"同质化"。

4.1.3　制订科学化培训方案

根据专业、等级和业务范围，有序分批分类对医院所有职工进行培训。为提高培训效率，培训分为理论自学和现场操作两个阶段，学员在参加现场培训前必须完成理论自学。现场培训采用课前测试、观看教学视频、导师分步讲授、模拟实战演练以及课后复测反馈的形式进行，力求使培训对象在培训结束后能够直接将所学技能应用于实践。

4.1.4 实施多角度课程评估

医院一方面定期收集导师和学员的培训反馈信息，另一方面则通过学员培训前后的技能测试，了解培训中存在的问题和不足，收集学员的潜在培训需求和建议，从而进一步优化培训内容，提高培训质量和效果。见图4-1。

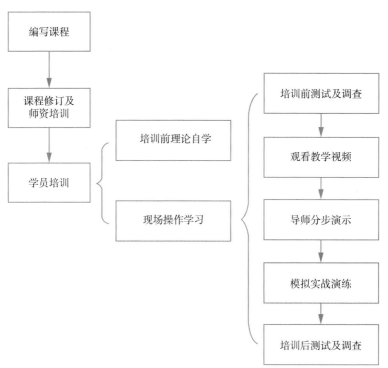

图4-1 医务人员培训流程

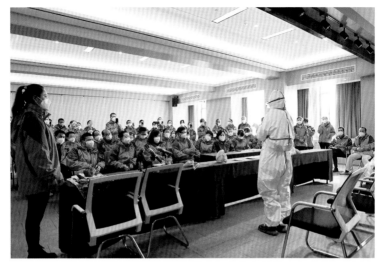

图4-2 受邀支持卓尔长江应急医院的西安国际医学中心医院援汉医疗队岗前培训

4.2 患者收治

4.2.1 预检分诊

预检分诊通过全面监测所有门诊进出人员，对高风险患者进行早期甄别，及时引导其到发热门诊就诊，防止交叉感染。三级分诊体系如下：

（1）第1级分诊

门诊设立发热患者预检分诊通道，红外体温枪监测所有进入人员体温，发现发热患者（体温超过37.3℃）立即用水银体温计复测腋温，同时询问流行病学史。若复测体温仍大于37.3℃，无论是否有流行病学史，均由分诊人员陪同前往发热门诊就诊。

（2）第2级分诊

门诊各护士站设体温监测点，对所有就诊患者监测体温，及时筛查发现发热病例，同时询问流行病学史。若有流行病学史，由诊区护士陪送到发热门诊；若无流行病学史，指导患者前往发热门诊就诊，排除后返回门诊就诊。

（3）第3级分诊

门诊医师接诊患者时应询问患者有无发热，有发热者，询问其流行病学史。对有流行病学史者，立即告知诊区护士，由诊区护士陪送到发热门诊；若无流行病学史，指导患者前往发热门诊就诊，排除后返回门诊就诊。

4.2.2 患者收治流程

医院首先通过发热门诊对患者进行实验室检查、影像学检查和流行病学调查，对非疑似病例进行一般治疗并嘱其居家隔离观察，对疑似病例则进行单人间隔离治疗并开展核酸检测；进一步，如间隔24小时两次核酸检测结果呈阴性，则对患者进行一般治疗并嘱其居家隔离观察；如核酸检测呈阳性，则根据症状和检查结果对患者进行分型，将轻症患者转至方舱医院进行隔离治疗，危重症患者留院隔离治疗；患者经治疗达到出院标准后，则转至"康复驿站"（患者接受康复治疗和医学观察的隔离点）进行14天的隔离观察和健康监测。

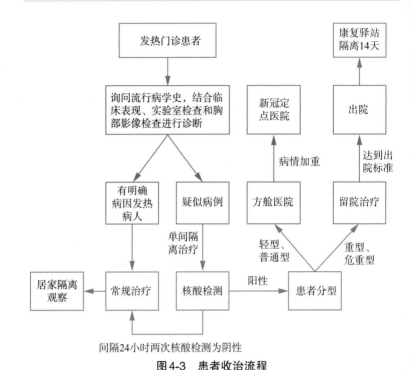

图4-3 患者收治流程

4.2.3 患者诊断标准

（1）新冠肺炎疑似患者诊断标准

结合下述流行病学史和临床表现综合分析，有流行病学史中的任何一条，且符合临床表现中任意2条；无明确流行病学史的，符合临床表现中的3条。

1）流行病学史

（a）发病前14天内有疫区及周边地区，或其他有病例报告地区的旅行史或居住史。

（b）发病前14天内与新型冠状病毒感染者（核酸检测呈阳性者）有接触史。

（c）发病前14天内曾接触过来自疫区及周边地区，或来自有病例报告地区的发热或有呼吸道症状的患者。

（d）聚集性发病（2周内在小范围，如家庭、办公室、学校、班级等场所，出现2例及以上发热和/或呼吸道症状的病例）。

2）临床表现

（a）发热和/或呼吸道症状。

（b）具有新型冠状病毒肺炎影像学特征。

（c）发病早期白细胞总数正常或降低，淋巴细胞计数正常或减少。

疑似病例连续两次新型冠状病毒核酸检测呈阴性（采样时间至少间隔24小时）且发病7天后新型冠状病毒特异性抗体IgM和IgG仍为阴性可排除疑似病例诊断。

（2）新冠肺炎确诊患者诊断标准

疑似病例同时具备以下病原学或血清学证据之一者即可确诊：

1）实时荧光RTPCR检测新型冠状病毒核酸呈阳性。

2）病毒基因测序，与已知的新型冠状病毒高度同源。

3）血清新型冠状病毒特异性IgM抗体和IgG抗体阳性；血清新型冠状病毒特异性IgG抗体由阴性转为阳性或恢复期较急性期4倍及以上升高。

（3）新冠肺炎确诊患者临床分型标准

1）轻型。临床症状轻微，影像学未见肺炎表现。

2）普通型。具有发热、呼吸道等症状，影像学可见肺炎表现。

3）重型。成人符合下列任何一条：

（a）出现气促，RR≥30次/分。

（b）静息状态下，指血氧饱和度≤93%。

（c）动脉血氧分压（PaO_2）/吸氧浓度（FiO_2）≤300mmHg（1mmHg＝0.133kPa）。

高海拔（海拔超过1000米）地区应根据以下公式对PaO_2/FiO_2进行校正：PaO_2/FiO_2×[大气压（mmHg）/760]。

肺部影像学显示24～48小时内病灶明显进展＞50%者按重型管理。

儿童符合下列任何一条：

（a）出现气促（＜2月龄，RR≥60次/分；2月龄至12月龄，RR≥50次/分；1岁至5岁，RR≥40次/分；＞5岁，RR≥30次/分），除外发热和哭闹的影响。

（b）静息状态下，指血氧饱和度≤92%。

（c）辅助呼吸（呻吟、鼻翼扇动、三凹征），发绀，间歇性呼吸暂停。

（d）出现嗜睡、惊厥。

（e）拒食或喂养困难，有脱水征。

4）危重型。符合以下情况之一者：

（a）出现呼吸衰竭，且需要机械通气。

（b）出现休克。

（c）合并其他器官功能衰竭需ICU监护治疗。

4.2.4　患者临床治疗

疑似病例应单人单间隔离治疗，确诊病例可多人收治在同一病室，危重型病例应当尽早收入ICU治疗。

患者治疗及护理严格按照政府最新发布的《新型冠状病毒肺炎诊疗方案》《新冠肺炎重型、危重型患者护理规范》《新冠肺炎重型、危重型患者治疗指南》等来操作执行。

4.2.5　患者心理干预策略

新冠肺炎的传播特点以及危害性，疫情暴发后医疗资源的相对不足以及其他社会因素，都会给新冠肺炎疑似及确诊患者带来较大的心理压力，进而对患者治疗过程和效果产生影响。因此，对新冠肺炎疑似和确诊患者进行心理干预是十分必要的。

（1）确诊患者

1）隔离治疗初期患者

患者心态：麻木、否认、愤怒、恐惧、焦虑、抑郁、失望、抱怨、失眠或攻击等。

干预原则：支持、安慰为主。宽容对待患者，稳定患者情绪，及早评估自杀、自伤、攻击风险。

干预措施：

（a）理解患者出现的情绪反应属于正常的应激反应，做到事先有所准备，不被患者的攻击和悲伤行为所激怒而失去医生的立场，如与患者争吵或过度卷入等。

（b）在理解患者的前提下，除药物治疗外应当给予心理危机干预，如及时评估自杀、自伤、攻击风险、正面心理支持、不与患者正面冲突等。必要时请精神科会诊。解释隔离治疗的重要性和必要性，鼓励患者树立积极恢复的信心。

（c）强调隔离手段不仅是为了更好地观察治疗患者，同时是保护亲人和社会安全的方式。解释目前治疗的要点和干预的有效性。

2）隔离治疗期患者

患者心态：除上述可能出现的心态以外，还可能出现孤独，或因对疾病的恐惧而不配合、放弃治疗，或对治疗的过度乐观和期望值过高等。

干预原则：积极沟通信息，必要时请精神科会诊。

干预措施：

（a）根据患者能接受的程度，客观如实交代病情和外界疫情，使患者做到心中有数。

（b）协助与外界亲人沟通，转达信息。

（c）积极鼓励患者配合治疗的所有行为。

（d）尽量使环境适宜患者的治疗。

（e）必要时请精神科会诊。

3）发生呼吸窘迫、极度不安、表达困难的患者

患者心态：濒死感、恐慌、绝望等。

干预原则：安抚、镇静，注意情感交流，增强治疗信心。

干预措施：镇定、安抚的同时，加强原发病的治疗，减轻症状。

（2）到医院就诊的发热患者

患者心态：恐慌、不安、孤独、无助、压抑、抑郁、悲观、愤怒、紧张，被他人疏远躲避的压力、委屈、羞耻感或不重视疾病等。

干预原则：健康宣教，鼓励配合、顺应变化。

干预措施：

（a）协助服务对象了解真实可靠的信息与知识，取信科学和医学权威资料。

（b）鼓励积极配合治疗和隔离措施，健康饮食和作息，多进行读书、听音乐、利用现代通信手段沟通及其他日常活动。

（c）接纳隔离处境，了解自己的反应，寻找逆境中的积极意义。

（d）寻求应对压力的社会支持：利用现代通信手段联络

亲朋好友、同事等，倾诉感受，保持与社会的沟通，获得支持鼓励。

（e）鼓励使用心理援助热线或在线心理干预等。

（3）疑似患者

患者心态：侥幸心理、躲避治疗、怕被歧视，或焦躁、过度求治、频繁转院等。

干预原则：及时宣教、正确防护、服从大局、减少压力。

干预措施：

（a）政策宣教、密切观察、及早求治。

（b）为人为己采用必要的保护措施。

（c）服从大局安排，按照规定报告个人情况。

（d）使用减压行为，减少应激。

4.2.6　患者出院标准

患者满足以下所有条件则可出院。见图4-4。

（1）体温恢复正常3天以上。

（2）呼吸道症状明显好转。

（3）肺部影像学显示急性渗出性病变明显改善。

（4）连续两次痰、鼻咽拭子等呼吸道标本核酸检测呈阴性（采样时间至少间隔24小时）。

患者出院后，应转至"康复驿站"继续进行14天的隔离管理。佩戴口罩，减少与他人近距离接触。加强营养，多喝水（每天3000ml以上），并逐渐进行室内活动。出院后第2周和第4周到医院随访和复诊。

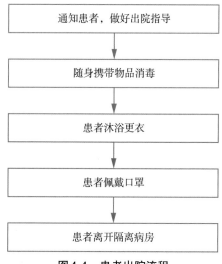

图 4-4　患者出院流程

4.3　医疗管理制度

4.3.1　发热门诊管理

（1）运营及人员配置：发热门诊 24 小时开放，由急诊科进行统一管理，指定经培训过的，有一定临床经验的医师负责组织对可疑病例的筛查、会诊、转诊、报告等工作。每个发热门诊每班由两名医生同时坐诊，并配备两名护士于清洁区辅助，此外每个发热门诊外再配置一名护士对相关工作进行协调处置。

（2）建筑布局：按照"三区两通道"划分，保证人员"单进单出"。

（3）留观室或抢救室加强通风，如使用机械通风，应当控制气流方向，由清洁侧流向污染侧。

（4）医务人员应当掌握新型冠状病毒感染的流行病学特点

与临床特征，按照诊疗规范进行患者筛查，对疑似或确诊患者立即采取隔离措施并及时报告。

（5）医疗机构应当为患者及陪同人员提供口罩并指导其正确佩戴。

4.3.2 病房管理

（1）对疑似或确诊患者应当及时采取隔离措施，疑似患者和确诊患者应当分开安置。疑似患者进行单间隔离，经病原学确诊的患者可以同室安置。

（2）进出隔离病房正确实施手卫生及穿脱防护用品。

（3）制定医务人员穿脱防护用品的流程，制作流程图和配置穿衣镜。配备熟练感染防控技术的人员督导医务人员防护用品的穿脱，防止污染。

（4）用于诊疗疑似或确诊患者的听诊器、体温计、血压计等医疗器具及护理物品应当专人专用。若条件有限，不能保障医疗器具专人专用时，每次使用后应当进行规范的清洁和消毒。

（5）重症患者应当收治在重症监护病房或者具备监护和抢救条件的病室，收治重症患者的监护病房或者具备监护和抢救条件的病室不得收治其他患者。

（6）严格探视制度，原则上不设陪护。若患者病情危重等特殊情况必须探视的，探视者必须严格按照规定做好个人防护。

（7）加强病室通风换气，每日用循环风空气消毒机进行空气消毒2次。

（8）确诊病例使用过的床单、被套、枕套用双层医疗废物袋盛装，袋外贴上"新型冠状病毒感染"字样，送至浆洗消毒供应中心消毒；枕芯、被褥、垫絮用床单元消毒机进行消毒，如有可见的血液等体液污染，按照感染性废物处理。

（9）传染病患者的生活垃圾按医疗废物进行处理。

（10）每日对医务人员的体温和症状进行监测，如有发热或出现呼吸道症状则立即报告医院感染管理部门。

4.3.3　患者管理

（1）对疑似或确诊患者及时进行隔离，并按照指定规范路线由专人引导进入隔离区。

（2）患者进入病区前更换患者服，个人物品及换下的衣服集中消毒处理后，存放于指定地点由医疗机构统一保管。

（3）指导患者正确选择、佩戴口罩，正确实施咳嗽礼仪和手卫生。

（4）加强对患者探视或陪护人员的管理。

（5）对被隔离的患者，原则上其活动限制在隔离病房内，减少患者的移动和转换病房，若确需离开隔离病房或隔离区域时，应当采取相应措施，如佩戴医用外科口罩，防止患者对其他患者和环境造成污染。

（6）疑似或确诊患者出院、转院时，更换干净衣服后方可离开，医务人员需对其接触环境进行终末消毒。

（7）疑似或确诊患者死亡的，对尸体应当及时进行处理。处理方法为：用3000mg/L的含氯消毒剂或0.5%过氧乙酸棉球或纱布填塞患者口、鼻、耳、肛门等所有开放通道；用双层布单包裹尸体，装入双层尸体袋中，由专用车辆直接送至指定地点火化。患者住院期间使用的个人物品经消毒后方可随患者家属带回家。

4.3.4　ICU病区设置与护理人力管理

（1）病区设置

应因地制宜、合理布局，严格划分污染区、潜在污染区和清洁区。在污染区、潜在污染区和清洁区之间设立缓冲区。各区域张贴醒目标识，防止误入。同时，设置医务人员通道和患者通道，确保不交叉。

（2）设备设施

1）急救物品及药品：配备一定数量的急救车及急救药品、氧气筒及配套装置、心电监护仪、心电图机、除颤仪、注射泵、输液泵、气管插管用物、便携式负压吸引器、无创呼吸机、有创呼吸机、血滤机及ECMO等设备。

2）消毒设备：空气消毒机、床单位消毒机、空气净化器、喷壶等。

3）气体及负压设备：准备足够压力的壁氧系统、压缩空气。

4）其他设施：冰箱、治疗车、轮椅、平车等。

（3）护理人力配置与排班原则

1）按照床护比1∶6配置护理人力，建议每班次4小时，合理排班。

2）护士应具有ICU专业背景，有较强的业务能力和较高的职业素质。

3）身体健康，能承担高强度医疗救治工作。

4.3.5　病例转运

（1）转运要求

1）转运救护车辆车载医疗设备（包括担架）专车专用，驾驶室与车厢严格密封隔离，车内设专门的污染物品放置区域，配备防护用品、消毒液、快速手消毒剂。

2）医务人员穿工作服、隔离衣，戴手套、工作帽、医用防护口罩；司机穿工作服，戴外科口罩、手套。

3）医务人员、司机转运新型冠状病毒感染的肺炎患者后，须及时更换全套防护物品。

4）转运救护车应具备转运呼吸道传染病患者基本条件，尽可能使用负压救护车进行转运。转运时应保持密闭状态，转运后对车辆进行消毒处理。转运重症病例时，应随车配备必要的生命支持设备，防止患者在转运过程中病情进一步恶化。

5）医务人员和司机的防护，车辆、医疗用品及设备消毒，污染物品处理等应严格按照标准执行。

6）救护车返回后需严格消毒方可再转运下一例患者。

（2）转运分级及配置

由专职住院总医师或当天值班二线医师根据患者转运前的情况及需要支持的手段决定转运级别，确定转运人员及准备的物品。根据所需器官功能支持的级别，将转运分为初级、中级、高级、相对禁忌和绝对禁忌5个等级。

1）初级：仅需要面罩吸氧即能转运的患者，使用低剂量升压药［多巴胺＜$5\mu g/$（$kg\cdot min$）或去甲肾上腺素＜$0.1\mu g/$（$kg\cdot min$）］；转运人员需原科室治疗的医生及护士各一名。

2）中级：需要机械通气的患者或使用中等剂量的升压药［多巴胺$510\mu g/$（$kg\cdot min$）或去甲肾上腺素$0.1\sim0.5\mu g/$（$kg\cdot min$）］；转运人员需重症医学科医生一名、呼吸治疗师（RT）和护士各一名。

3）高级：机械通气支持力度高［吸氧浓度$60\%\sim80\%$，呼气末正压（PEEP）$10\sim12cmH_2O$（$1cmH_2O\approx0.098kPa$）］；高剂量血管活性药［多巴胺$10\sim15\mu g/$（$kg\cdot min$）或去甲肾上腺素$0.5\sim1.0\mu g/$（$kg\cdot min$）］；ECMO支持的患者。转运人员需科室住院总医师或值班二线一名、RT和护士各一名，或ECMO转运团队。

4）转运相对禁忌：生命体征极不稳定或内环境极度紊乱，随时面临心搏骤停抢救的状态；机械通气支持力度很高（吸氧浓度≥80%，PEEP≥10cmH$_2$O）；超大剂量血管活性药物〔多巴胺≥15μg/（kg·min）或去甲肾上腺素≥1μg/（kg·min）〕；建议就地抢救，待生命体征稍稳定后再进行转运。

5）转运绝对禁忌：正在实施心肺复苏及实施心肺复苏后在极高水平支持下呼吸循环状态仍不稳定（SpO$_2$＜90%，SBP＜90mmHg）。

（3）转运流程

穿、戴防护物品→出车至医疗机构接患者→患者戴外科口罩→将患者安置在救护车→将患者转运至接收医疗机构→车辆及设备消毒→转运下一例患者。

（4）穿戴及脱摘防护物品流程

穿戴防护物品流程：洗手或手消毒→戴帽子→戴医用防护口罩→穿工作服→穿隔离衣→戴手套。

脱摘防护物品流程：摘手套→洗手或手消毒→脱隔离衣→洗手或手消毒→摘口罩帽子→洗手或手消毒。

医务人员、司机下班前进行手卫生→淋浴更衣。

（5）救护车清洁消毒

1）空气：开窗通风。

2）车厢及其物体表面：用过氧化氢喷雾或含氯消毒剂擦拭消毒。

4.3.6 医务人员防护

（1）医疗机构和医务人员应当强化标准预防措施的落实，做好诊区、病区（房）的通风管理，佩戴医用外科口罩/医用防护口罩，必要时戴乳胶手套。

（2）采取飞沫隔离、接触隔离和空气隔离防护措施，根据不同情形，做到以下防护：

1）接触患者的血液、体液、分泌物、排泄物、呕吐物及污染物品时：戴清洁手套，脱手套后洗手。

2）可能受到患者血液、体液、分泌物等喷溅时：戴医用防护口罩、护目镜，穿防渗隔离衣。

3）为疑似患者或确诊患者实施可能产生气溶胶的操作（如气管插管、无创通气、气管切开，心肺复苏，插管前手动通气和支气管镜检查等）时：

（a）采取空气隔离措施。

（b）佩戴医用防护口罩，并进行密闭性能检测。

（c）眼部防护（如佩戴护目镜或面罩）。

（d）穿防体液渗入的长袖隔离衣，戴手套。

（e）操作应当在通风良好的房间内进行。

（f）房间中人数限制在患者所需护理和支持的最低数量。

（3）医务人员使用的防护用品应当符合国家有关标准。

（4）医用外科口罩、医用防护口罩、护目镜、隔离衣等防护用品被患者血液、体液、分泌物等污染时应当及时更换。

（5）正确使用防护用品，戴手套前应当洗手，脱去手套或隔离服后应当立即用流动水洗手。

（a）外科口罩：预检分诊、发热门诊及全院诊疗区域应当使用，需正确佩戴。污染或潮湿时随时更换。

（b）医用防护口罩：原则上在发热门诊、隔离留观病区（房）、隔离病区（房）和隔离重症监护病区（房）等区域，以及进行采集呼吸道标本、气管插管、气管切开、无创通气、吸痰等可能产生气溶胶的操作时使用。一般4小时更换一次，污染或潮湿时随时更换。其他区域和在其他区域的诊疗操作，原则上不使用。

（c）乳胶检查手套：在预检分诊、发热门诊、隔离留观病区（房）、隔离病区（房）和隔离重症监护病区（房）等区域使用，但需正确穿戴和脱摘，注意及时更换手套。禁止戴手套离开诊疗区域。戴手套不能取代手卫生。

（d）速干手消毒剂：医务人员诊疗操作过程中，手部未见明显污染物时使用，全院均应当使用。预检分诊、发热门诊、隔离留观病区（房）、隔离病区（房）和隔离重症监护病区（房）必须配备使用。

（e）护目镜：在隔离留观病区（房）、隔离病区（房）和隔离重症监护病区（房）等区域，以及采集呼吸道标本、气管插管、气管切开、无创通气、吸痰等可能出现血液、体液和分泌物等喷溅操作时使用。禁止戴着护目镜离开上述区域。如护目镜为可重复使用的，应当消毒后再复用。其他区域和在其他区域的诊疗操作原则上不使用护目镜。

（f）防护面罩/防护面屏：诊疗操作中可能发生血液、体液和分泌物等喷溅时使用。如为可重复使用的，使用后应当消毒方可再用；如为一次性使用的，不得重复使用。禁止戴着防护面罩/防护面屏离开诊疗区域。

（g）隔离衣：预检分诊、发热门诊使用普通隔离衣，隔离留观病区（房）、隔离病区（房）和隔离重症监护病区（房）使用防渗一次性隔离衣，其他科室或区域根据是否接触患者使用。一次性隔离衣不得重复使用。如使用可复用的隔离衣，使用后按规定消毒后方可再用。禁止穿着隔离衣离开上述区域。

（h）防护服：隔离留观病区（房）、隔离病区（房）和隔离重症监护病区（房）使用。防护服不得重复使用。禁止戴着医用防护口罩和穿着防护服离开上述区域。其他区域和在其他区域的诊疗操作原则上不使用防护服。

4.3.7 穿脱防护用品流程

（1）医务人员进入隔离病区穿戴防护用品

（清洁区进入潜在污染区前）

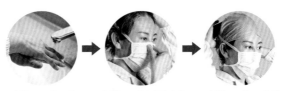

步骤1：手卫生　　步骤2：戴医用防护　　步骤3：戴一次性
　　　　　　　　　口罩（N95及以上）　　　　工作帽

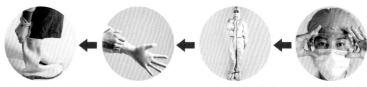

步骤7：穿防水靴　步骤6：戴里层　　步骤5：穿一次性　步骤4：戴防护
　　　　　　　　一次性手套　　　　防护服　　　　　眼罩

（潜在污染区进入污染区前）

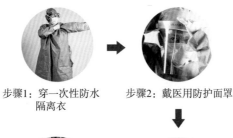

步骤1：穿一次性防水　　步骤2：戴医用防护面罩
　　　　隔离衣

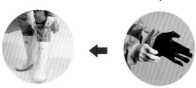

步骤4：换一次性靴套　　步骤3：戴外层手套

图4-5　医务人员进入隔离病区穿戴防护用品流程

（2）医务人员离开隔离病区脱摘防护用品

（污染区回到潜在污染区前）

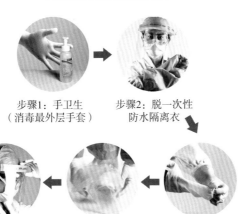

步骤1：手卫生　　步骤2：脱一次性
（消毒最外层手套）　　防水隔离衣

步骤5：消毒内层　步骤4：消毒内层手套　步骤3：脱外层
手套后摘防护面罩　后脱一次性靴套　一次性乳胶手套

（潜在污染区回到清洁区前）

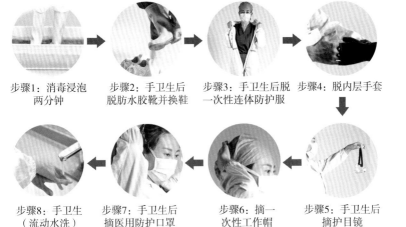

步骤1：消毒浸泡　步骤2：手卫生后　步骤3：手卫生后脱　步骤4：脱内层手套
两分钟　脱防水胶靴并换鞋　一次性连体防护服

步骤8：手卫生　步骤7：手卫生后　步骤6：摘一　步骤5：手卫生后
（流动水洗）　摘医用防护口罩　次性工作帽　摘护目镜

图4-6　医务人员离开隔离病区脱摘防护用品流程

（3）一次性外科口罩的佩戴与脱卸

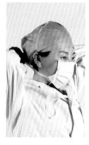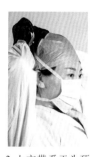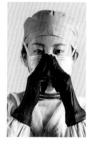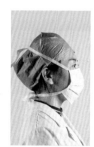

1. 口罩罩住鼻、口及下巴，口罩下方带系于颈后

2. 上方带系于头顶中部

3. 将双手指尖放于鼻夹上，从中间位置开始，用手指向内按压，并逐步向两侧移动，根据鼻梁形状塑造鼻夹

4. 调整系带松紧度，使其贴合面部

图4-7　戴一次性外科口罩流程

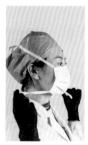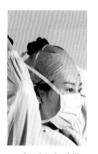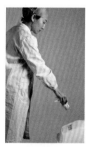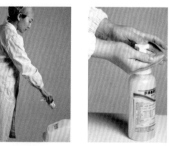

1. 不接触口罩前面，先解开下方系带

2. 解开上方系带

3. 用手捏住系带投入医疗废弃物袋中

4. 手卫生

图4-8　脱一次性外科口罩流程

（4）医用防护口罩佩戴及脱卸

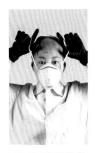 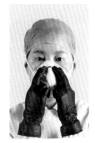 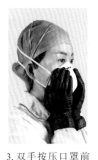 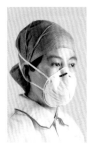

1.防护口罩罩住鼻、口及下巴，鼻尖部紧贴面部。两手拉着口罩的松紧带，拉过头顶，放在颈后和头中部

2.将双手指尖放在金属鼻夹上，从中间位置开始，用手指向内按鼻夹，并分别向两侧移动和按压，根据鼻梁的形状塑造鼻夹

3.双手按压口罩前部并进行正压密合性实验：大口呼气，出现正压表明无漏气；如果漏气，调整口罩位置或收紧带子

4.进行负压密合性实验：深吸气，如不漏气，口罩将紧贴面部；如果漏气，调整口罩位置或收紧带子

图4-9　医用防护口罩佩戴流程

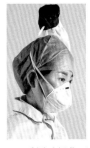 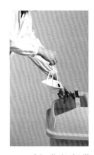 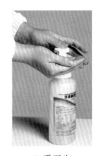

1.双手同时抓住两根松紧带，提过头部，脱下

2.双手捏住松紧带投入医疗废弃袋中

3.手卫生

图4-10　医用防护口罩脱卸流程

（5）隔离衣穿戴和脱卸

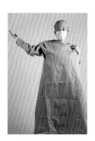 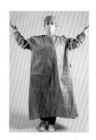 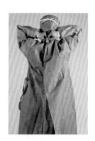

1. 左手提衣领，右手伸入袖内，左手将衣领向上拉，漏出右手

2. 换右手持衣领，左手伸入袖内，漏出右手，勿触及面部

3. 两手持衣领，由领子中央顺着边缘向后系好颈带

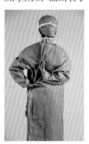 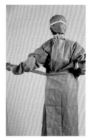 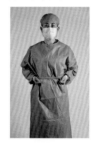

4. 双手在背后将衣边对齐

5. 向一侧折叠，一手按住折叠处，另一手将腰带拉至背后折叠处

6. 将腰带在背后交叉，回到前面将带子系好

图4-11　穿隔离衣流程

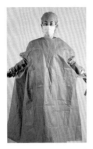 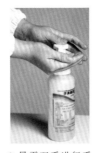 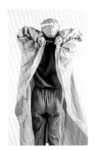

1. 解开腰带，在前面打一个活结

2. 暴露双手进行手消毒

3. 解颈后带子

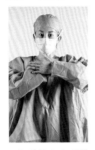 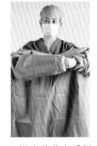 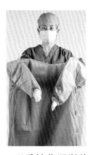

4. 右手伸入左手腕部袖子内，拉下袖子过手

5. 用遮盖着左手握住右手隔离衣袖子的外面，拉下右侧袖子

6. 双手转化逐渐从袖管退出，脱下隔离衣

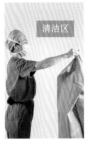 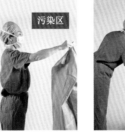

7. 左手握住领子，右手将隔离衣两边对齐，如挂在污染区，则污染面向外，如挂于污染区外，则污染面向里

8. 不再使用时，将脱下的隔离衣，污染面向内，卷成包囊状，丢至指定回收处

图4-12　脱隔离衣流程

（6）连体式防护衣穿戴和脱卸

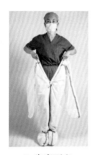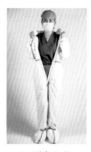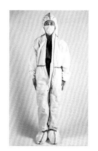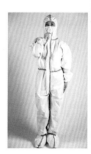

1. 先穿下衣　　　2. 再穿上衣　　　3. 戴好帽子　　　4. 拉好拉链

图4-13　穿连体式防护衣流程

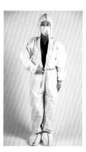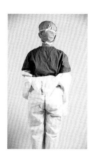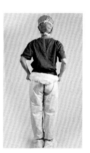

1. 将拉链拉至底　　　2. 脱下袖子　　　3. 由上向下边脱边卷防护衣，污染面向里，将污染面向里卷成包裹状，丢至医疗废物容器

图4-14　脱连体式防护衣流程

（7）护目镜或防护面罩佩戴及脱卸

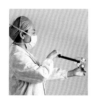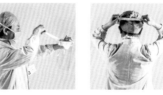

1. 检查有无破损，佩戴装置有无松懈　　　2. 抓住护目镜或者防护面罩的耳围或头围带上，调节舒适度

图4-15　戴护目镜或防护面罩流程

1.抓住护目镜的耳围或者防护面罩的头围 末端,摘掉护目镜

2.可重复使用的,放在带盖容器内集中清 洁消毒;不可重复使用的,丢入黄色医疗 废物垃圾桶,随后手卫生

图4-16 脱护目镜或防护面罩流程

4.3.8 防护物资配置

（1）暴露风险级别分区

根据不同的暴露风险级别,将恢复日常诊疗工作的医务人员分别采取不同的个人防护措施。

1）高风险暴露区域:直接或可能接触患者或患者的污染物及其污染物品和环境表面的所有医务人员。具体科室包括重症监护室、急诊科、预检分诊、发热门诊、急诊外科手术、检验科、产房、导管室和透析室等侵入性操作科室。

2）低风险暴露区域:直接接触患者或患者的污染物及其污染物品和环境表面概率较低的人员。具体包括普通门诊、普通病房、医技科室、一线管理人员以及工勤人员（保洁、轮换库、安保、食堂、太平间、医疗废弃物处置人员、陪护人员等）。

（2）配置标准

原则上按不同风险暴露级别和不同岗位要求,配置不同的医用防护物资。

1）高风险暴露区域

配备品目:医用防护服、医用防护口罩、护目镜或防护面罩、隔离衣、一次性外科口罩、一次性工作帽、一次性医用

手套。

配备标准：重症监护室、急诊外科手术、检验科、产房、导管室和透析室等侵入性操作科室在所有急诊入院未完成新冠肺炎排查的患者诊疗时，医务人员必须配备医用防护服、医用防护口罩、护目镜或防护面罩、一次性工作帽、一次性医用手套。

2）低风险暴露区域

配备品目：医用防护口罩或医用外科口罩、一次性工作帽、一次性医用手套、工作服或隔离衣。

配备标准：医疗机构全口径人员配备。

第五章　新冠应急医院后勤保障

5.1　物资储备与保障

5.1.1　常用物资储备

（1）常用药品

目前，尚无确认有效的抗病毒治疗药物和方法，比较常用的药物和用法有以下几种：

1）α-干扰素：成人每次500万国际单位或相当剂量，加入灭菌注射用水2ml，每日2次雾化吸入。

2）洛匹那韦/利托那韦：成人每粒200mg/50mg，每次2粒，每日2次，疗程不超过10天。

3）利巴韦林：建议与干扰素或洛匹那韦/利托那韦联合应用，成人500mg/次，每日2次至3次静脉输注，疗程不超过10天。

4）阿比多尔：成人200mg，每日3次，疗程不超过10天。

5）磷酸氯喹：成人500mg，每日2次，疗程不超过10天。

除上述药品外，抗病毒、抗菌、解热镇痛、止咳平喘化痰、胃肠、肠道微生态调节剂、免疫力调节等药品对治疗新冠肺炎亦有促进作用。

根据新冠应急医院收治情况，结合以上药品用量，合理储备。

（2）常用设备

检测设备：红外线测温仪、PCR 检测仪、监护仪等。

治疗设备：呼吸机、制氧机、除颤仪、注射泵等。

消毒设备：测温灭菌站、紫外线消毒灯等。

（3）常用防护用品

新冠应急医院的常用防护用品主要有：工作帽、外科口罩、医用防护口罩（N95）、工作服、一次性医用防护服、高级防护服、一次性乳胶手套、全面型呼吸防护器、正压式头套、护目镜、一次性隔离衣、防护鞋（靴）、消毒液等。

5.1.2　物资采购供应

新冠应急医院负责制定药品、防护用品及设备需求表，公益机构统一采购。在保障常用药物供给的基础上，重点保障应对 COVID-19 防治相关药物的供给。物资采购必须从有合法资质的药品经营企业购入，将有关经营企业和业务人员的资质进行备案。发生物资短缺时应积极与供货商协商沟通，督促其扩大进货渠道或以区域间调货等方式予以解决。存在采购困难的，应积极征询医院建议寻找替代物资。

5.1.3　药品捐赠

接受捐赠药品的标准：

1）境内生产的药品，必须是经当地药品监管部门批准生产、获得批准文号且符合质量标准的品种，有效期限距失效日期须在 6 个月以上。

2）境外生产的药品，应是当地药品监管部门批准注册的品种，以及国际上通用药典收载、在注册国合法生产并上市且符合质量标准的品种，有效期限距失效日期须在 12 个月以上；药品批准有效期为12个月及以下的，有效期限距失效日期须在6个月以上。

5.2 仓储物流保障

为提高管理效率和资源使用效率，所有新冠应急医院的医疗、生活物资施行统一管理，集中存放，并组建专业运输队，根据各新冠应急医院实际需求进行及时调配。见图5-1、图5-2。

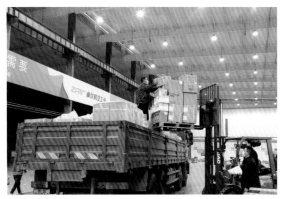

图5-1 卓尔应急医院仓库

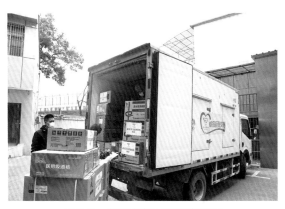

图5-2 卓尔应急医院物资调配

5.2.1 仓库管理制度

（1）职责

1）负责物资的收货、入库、发货、退货、储存、防护工作。

2）负责物资装卸、搬运、包装等工作。

3）负责废弃物品处理工作。

（2）管理要求

1）根据每批物资的到货情况，清点无误后制作入库单据予以入库管理。

2）按照物资分配要求，对接新冠应急医院提货人与运输车辆，清点无误后制作出库单并由提货人签字出库。

3）每天对暂未分配的物资进行盘点，制作库存表、物资流向表等，并对物资进行妥善分类保存。

5.2.2 运输管理制度

听从指挥、统一调度，制定合理运输方案，安全、快速地将物资运送至新冠应急医院。

5.3 膳食营养保障

5.3.1 膳食营养方案

（1）普通型或康复期患者的营养膳食

1）能量要充足，每天摄入谷薯类食物250～400克，包括大米、面粉、杂粮等；保证充足蛋白质，主要摄入优质蛋白质类食物（每天150～200克），如瘦肉、鱼、虾、蛋、大豆等，尽量保证每天一个鸡蛋，300克的奶及奶制品（酸奶能提供肠道益生菌，可多选）；通过多种烹调植物油增加必需脂肪酸的摄入，特别是单不饱和脂肪酸的植物油，总脂肪供能比达到膳食总能量的25%～30%。

2）多吃新鲜蔬菜和水果。蔬菜每天500克以上，水果每天200～350克，多选深色蔬果。

3）保证充足饮水量。每天1500～2000毫升，多次少量，主要饮白开水或淡茶水。饭前饭后可喝菜汤、鱼汤、鸡汤等。

4）杜绝食用野生动物，少吃辛辣刺激性食物。

5）食欲较差进食不足者、老年人及慢性病患者，可以通过营养强化食品、特殊医学用途配方食品或营养素补充剂，适量补充蛋白质以及B族维生素和维生素A、维生素C、维生素D等微量营养素。

（2）重症型患者的营养治疗重症型患者常伴有食欲下降、进食不足，使原本较弱的抵抗力"雪上加霜"。要重视危重症患者的营养治疗。为此提出序贯营养支持治疗原则：

1）少量多餐，每日6～7次利于吞咽和消化的流质食物，以蛋、大豆及其制品、奶及其制品、果汁、蔬菜汁、米粉等食材为主，注意补充足量优质蛋白质。病情逐渐缓解的过程中，可摄入半流质状态、易于咀嚼和消化的食物，随病情好转逐步向普通膳食过渡。

2）如食物未能达到营养需求。可在医生或者临床营养师指导下，正确使用肠内营养制剂（特殊医学用途配方食品）。

3）在食物和肠内营养不足或者不能摄入的情况下，对于严重胃肠道功能障碍的患者，需采用肠外营养以保持基本营养需求。在早期阶段可以达到营养摄入量的60%～80%，病情减轻后再逐步补充能量及营养素达到全量。

4）患者营养方案应该根据机体总体情况、出入量、肝肾功能以及糖脂代谢情况而制定。

（3）一线工作者营养膳食指导

根据平衡膳食原则，一线工作者的营养膳食要做到以下几点。

1）保证每天足够的能量摄入。建议男性能量摄入2400～2700千卡/天、女性2100～2300千卡/天。

2）保证每天摄入优质蛋白质，如蛋类、奶类、畜禽肉类、鱼虾类、大豆类等。

3）饮食宜清淡，忌油腻，可用天然香料等进行调味以增加医务人员的食欲。

4）多吃富含B族维生素、维生素C、矿物质和膳食纤维的食物，合理搭配米面、蔬菜、水果等，多选择油菜、菠菜、芹菜、紫甘蓝、胡萝卜、西红柿及橙类、苹果、猕猴桃等深色蔬果以及菇类、木耳、海带等菌藻类食物。

5）尽可能每日饮水量达到1500～2000毫升。

6）工作忙碌、普通膳食摄入不足时，可补充性使用肠内营养制剂（特殊医学用途配方食品）和奶粉、营养素补充剂，每日额外口服营养补充能量400～600千卡，保证营养需求。

7）采用分餐制就餐，同时避免相互混合用餐，降低就餐过程的感染风险。

8）医院分管领导、营养科、膳食管理科等，应因地制宜、及时根据一线工作人员身体状况，合理设计膳食，做好营养保障。

5.3.2 餐饮配送

疫情发生后，新冠应急医院自身后勤很难满足患者和医务人员的餐饮需求。与此同时，由于防控需要，当地的餐饮行业可能会被迫减少或停止运营。在此情况下，公益机构应在与医院进行充分沟通的基础上，制定出膳食营养方案，并寻找符合要求的配餐机构供餐。以卓尔汉江应急医院为例，配餐机构借助专业的保温货车将餐食运抵隔离楼门口；随后，医院后勤保障组根据各病区上报的用餐数量，安排人员送至各病区的清洁区；最后，由值班护士领取后送进病房。

5.4 清洁与消毒

5.4.1 空气消毒

日常消毒：每日≥4次；接诊疑似及确诊患者后诊室随时消毒。

有人状态：①自然通风，每次30分钟；②循环风紫外线空气消毒，每次2小时。

无人状态：①可选用有人状态的室内空气消毒方法；②紫外线灯照射消毒，每次1小时。

终末消毒：在无人条件下可选择过氧乙酸、二氧化氯、过氧化氢等消毒剂，采用超低容量喷雾法进行消毒，消毒完毕，打开门窗彻底通风。

5.4.2 环境物表清洁消毒

日常消毒：每日≥4次。

随时消毒：接诊疑似及确诊患者后，给诊室及转运工具消毒。

终末消毒：每日工作结束后。

消毒方法：物表用1000mg/L的含氯消毒液擦拭或喷洒消

毒，作用30分钟后用清水擦拭干净；地面消毒用1000mg/L的含氯消毒液拖地，消毒作用时间应不少于30分钟。

5.4.3 地面墙面清洁消毒

用1000mg/L含氯消毒剂对走廊、卫生间、盥洗室、污物处置、医废暂存间等空间表面进行均匀喷洒消毒，作用30分钟，每日4次；用1000mg/L含氯消毒剂拖地，作用时间30分钟，每日4次。

5.4.4 医疗器械器具消毒

尽可能选用一次性医疗器械、器具，用后按医疗废物处理；可重复使用的医疗器械使用后，先用2000mg/L含氯消毒剂浸泡消毒30分钟，再用专用容器密闭回收并标注"新冠"，消毒供应中心首选压力蒸汽灭菌，不耐热物品可选择化学消毒剂或低温灭菌设备进行消毒或灭菌。

5.4.5 患者血液、排泄物、分泌物、呕吐物处理

（1）少量污染物可用一次性吸水材料（如纱布、抹布等）沾取5000～10000mg/L的含氯消毒液（或能达到高水平消毒的消毒湿巾/干巾）小心移除。

（2）大量污染物应使用含吸水成分的消毒粉或漂白粉完全覆盖，或用一次性吸水材料完全覆盖后用足量的5000～10000mg/L的含氯消毒液浇在吸水材料上，作用30分钟以上（或能达到高水平消毒的消毒干巾），小心清除干净。清除过程中避免接触污染物，清理的污染物按医疗废物集中处置。患者的排泄物、分泌物、呕吐物等应有专门容器收集，用20000mg/L含氯消毒剂，按物、药1∶2的比例浸泡消毒2小时。

（3）清除污染物后，应对污染的环境物体表面进行消毒。盛放污染物的容器可用含有效氯5000mg/L的消毒剂溶液浸泡消毒30分钟，然后清洗干净。

5.4.6　其他

（1）对于患者的餐具、剩饭、菜渣，应消毒处理。

（2）晨间护理时用一次性扫床套扫床，一床一套。患者的衣服、床单、被套、枕套污染后及时更换；床头柜、病床、椅子、凳子等每日用消毒液擦拭消毒，患者出院、死亡后，床单要进行终末消毒。

（3）患者被服等纺织品，在收集时应避免产生气溶胶，建议均按医疗废物集中焚烧处理；若需重复使用，先用2000mg/L的含氯消毒液浸泡30分钟，按常规清洗；用水溶性包装袋按感染性织物收集，交织物洗涤公司洗涤消毒；贵重衣物可选用环氧乙烷方法进行消毒处理。

5.5　医疗废物管理

5.5.1　医疗废物的分类收集

（1）明确分类收集范围。医疗机构在诊疗新型冠状病毒感染的肺炎患者及疑似患者发热门诊和病区（房）产生的废弃物，包括医疗废物和生活垃圾，均应当按照医疗废物进行分类收集。

（2）规范包装容器。医疗废物专用包装袋、利器盒的外表面应当有警示标识。在盛装医疗废物前，应当进行认真检查，确保其无破损、无渗漏。医疗废物收集桶宜为脚踏式并带盖。医疗废物达到包装袋或者利器盒的3/4时，应当有效封口，确保封口严密。应当使用双层包装袋盛装医疗废物，采用鹅颈结式封口，分层封扎。

（3）做好安全收集。按照医疗废物类别及时分类收集，确保人员安全，控制感染风险。盛装医疗废物的包装袋和利器盒的外表面被感染性废物污染时，应当增加一层包装袋。分类收集使用后的一次性隔离衣、防护服等物品时，严禁挤压。每个包装袋、利器盒应当系有或粘贴标签，标签内容包括：医疗废物产生单位、产生部门、产生日期、类别，并在特别说明中标注"新型冠状病毒感染肺炎"或者简写为"新冠"。

（4）分区域进行处理。收治新型冠状病毒感染的肺炎患者及疑似患者发热门诊和病区（房）的潜在污染区和污染区产生的医疗废物，在离开污染区前应当对包装袋表面采用1000mg/L的含氯消毒液喷洒消毒（注意喷洒均匀）或在其外面加套一层医疗废物包装袋；清洁区产生的医疗废物按照常规的医疗废物处置。

（5）做好病原标本处理。医疗废物中含病原体的标本和相关保存液等高危险废物，应当在产生地点进行压力蒸汽灭菌或者化学消毒处理，然后按照感染性废物收集处理。

5.5.2　医疗废物的运送贮存

（1）安全运送管理。在运送医疗废物前，应当检查包装袋或者利器盒的标识、标签以及封口是否符合要求。工作人员在运送医疗废物时，应当防止造成医疗废物专用包装袋和利器盒的破损，防止医疗废物直接接触身体，避免医疗废物泄漏和扩散。每天运送结束后，对运送工具进行清洁和消毒，含氯消毒液浓度为1000mg/L；运送工具被感染性医疗废物污染时，应当及时消毒处理。

（2）贮存交接管理。医疗废物暂存处应当有严密的封闭措施，设有工作人员进行管理，防止非工作人员接触医疗废物。医疗废物宜在暂存处单独设置区域存放，尽快交由医疗废物处置单位进行处置。用1000mg/L的含氯消毒液对医疗废物暂存处地面进行消毒，每天两次。医疗废物产生部门、运送人员、暂存处工作人员以及医疗废物处置单位转运人员之间，要逐层登记交接，并说明其来源于新型冠状病毒感染的肺炎患者或疑似患者。

5.5.3 医疗废物的处置

焚烧处置场所不得带入或存放与处置无关的物品和个人生活用品；焚烧作业时，医疗废物处于完好包装状态；焚烧完毕后，应对有关设备、容器及场所进行彻底的清洗和消毒；医疗废物处置设备维修、维护前应当做好消毒和清洗工作；医疗废物处置过程中产生的污水（包括消毒清洗运送工具、周转箱、暂时贮存设施、处置现场地面的污水）应当经污水集中处理设施消毒处理后方可排放。

5.6 人员关怀

由于工作风险高、工作强度大，医务人员往往面临心理压力大、生理负荷重的问题，这可能会影响其工作积极性和质量。在感染数量大，医疗资源相对不足的情况下，患者也容易出现消极懈怠等心理问题。因此有必要针对医务人员和患者制定一系列关怀和激励措施。见图5-3。

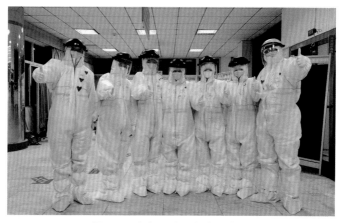

图5-3 应急医院医务人员合影

5.6.1 医务人员关怀

（1）改善医务人员工作和休息条件

加强医务人员职业暴露的防护设施建设和设备配置，尽可能为一线医务人员提供单人单间的休息场所，确保其休息和隔离需要，并做好饮食、基本生活用品等保障。

（2）合理安排医务人员作息时间

根据疫情防控实际，科学测算医务人员工作负荷，合理配置医务人员，在满足医疗服务需求的同时，保障医务人员休息时间。一线医务人员，原则上连续工作时间不得长于一个月；重症救治一线医务人员，连续工作时间可适当缩短；对于因执行疫情防控不能休假的医务人员，防控任务结束后，医疗机构优先安排补休。

（3）加强医务人员健康防护

尽一切可能配齐防护物资和防护设备，防护用品调配向临床一线倾斜。组织做好一线医务人员健康体检，有条件的要尽可能安排CT检查等。最大限度减少院内感染，发现医务人员感染及时隔离、全力救治。

（4）开展医务人员心理危机干预和心理疏导

在医疗机构内部成立由心理医师和其他医务人员组成的心理咨询自助工作队，开展医务人员心理健康评估，强化心理援助措施。开展以一线医务人员及其家属为重点的心理危机干预和日常心理疏导，减轻医务人员心理压力。对于发生应激症状的医务人员，及时安排换岗。

（5）强化对一线医务人员人文关怀

对一线医务人员及其家属开展慰问，定期了解他们的需求和困难，积极协调解决。

（6）实行人事人才倾斜政策

将医务人员在疫情防控工作中的表现作为人才评价和人事管理的重要依据，对作出贡献的医务人员在职称评审、人才项目评选和事业单位岗位聘用时予以倾斜，优先推荐、优先晋升。

（7）提高医务人员待遇

提高医务人员工资水平，为医务人员发放补助津贴。

（8）保障执业环境

加强安全保障，对歧视、孤立一线医务人员及其家属的行为进行批评教育；对在疫情防控工作中伤害医务人员、故意传播病原体、扰乱医疗秩序等行为进行依法处理。

（9）加强宣传表彰

对在疫情防控一线作出突出贡献的医疗卫生团队和个人，及时开展表彰奖励。

5.6.2　患者关怀

（1）开展患者心理危机干预和心理疏导

在医疗机构内部成立心理咨询自助工作队，开展患者心理健康评估，并进行心理危机干预和日常心理疏导，减轻患者心理压力。

（2）实施经济补助

为经济困难的患者提供一定经济补助，以鼓励其积极应对病情并配合治疗。

参考文献

［1］中华人民共和国住房和城乡建设部. GB 50849—2014传染病医院建筑设计规范［S］. 北京：中国计划出版社，2015.

［2］中华人民共和国住房和城乡建设部，中华人民共和国国家发展和改革委员会. 建标1732016传染病医院建设标准［S］. 北京：中国计划出版社，2016.

［3］中国工程建设标准化协会. 新型冠状病毒感染的肺炎传染病应急医疗设施设计标准［S］. 北京：中国建筑工业出版社，2020.

［4］浙江省住房和城乡建设厅，浙江省卫生和计划生育委员会. 浙江省传染病区（房）建筑设计标准［S］. 杭州：浙江省标准设计站，2006.

［5］浙江省住房和城乡建设厅. 浙江省传染病应急医院（呼吸类）建设技术导则（试行）［Z］. 2020.

［6］浙江省住房和城乡建设厅. 浙江省医院烈性传染病区（房）应急改造技术导则（试行）［Z］. 2020.

［7］中华人民共和国国家卫生和健康委员会，中华人民共和国住房和城乡建设部. 关于印发新型冠状病毒肺炎应急救治设施设计导则（试行）的通知［EB/OL］. http://www.gov.cn/zhengce/zhengceku/202002/11/content_5477301.htm

［8］四川大学华西医院，四川省新型冠状病毒感染肺炎医疗救治专家组. 新冠肺炎医疗机构紧急防控指南［M］. 成都：四川科学技术出版社，2020.

［9］中华人民共和国国务院. 关于依法科学精准做好新冠肺炎疫情防控工作的通知［EB/OL］. http://www.nhc.gov.cn/jkj/s3577/202002/69b3fd-cbb61f499ba50a25cdf1d5374e.shtml

［10］吕占秀，周先志，等. 现代传染病医院管理学［M］. 北京：人民军

医出版社，2010.

［11］黄刚，楼天正，等. 基层医院新型冠状病毒肺炎防治手册［M］. 杭州：浙江大学出版社，2020.

［12］中华人民共和国国家卫生和健康委员会. 新型冠状病毒感染的肺炎防治营养膳食指导［EB/OL］. http://www.nhc.gov.cn/xcs/yqfk-dt/202002/a69fd36d54514c5a9a3f456188cbc428.shtml

［13］胡必杰，刘荣辉，等. SIFIC 医院感染预防与控制操作图解［M］. 上海：上海科学技术出版社，2015.

［14］中华人民共和国国家卫生和健康委员会. 新型冠状病毒感染的肺炎疫情紧急心理危机干预指导原则［EB/OL］. http://www.nhc.gov.cn/jkj/s3577/202001/6adc08b966594253b2b791be5c3b9467.shtml

［15］湖北省卫生和健康委员会，教育厅，财政厅，人力资源和社会保障厅. 关于进一步关爱和激励新冠肺炎疫情防控一线医务人员的若干措施［EB/OL］. http://www.hubei.gov.cn/zfwj/ezbf/202002/t20200218_2103386.shtml

鸣　谢

马云公益基金会

阿里巴巴公益基金会

武汉市第八医院

武汉市汉阳医院

黄冈市中心医院

黄陂区人民医院盘龙城分院

罗田县第二人民医院

监利县人民医院

随州市中心医院

EMERGENCY HOSPITALS FOR COVID-19

CONSTRUCTION AND OPERATION MANUAL

Yan Zhi **Editor-in-Chief**

Yan Ge **English translator**

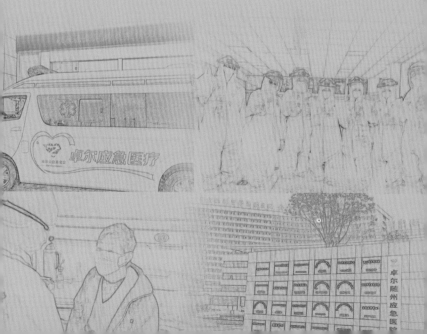

Editor-in-Chief: Yan Zhi

Contributors: Yan Zhi, Zhang Liang, Du Shuwei,
Tian Xudong, Niu Yadong,
Xiong Xiaochuan

English translator: Yan Ge

English proofreader: Wang Sida

Layout designers: Huang Xuan, Song Jie, Ye Qinyun,
Hu Yangfu

Photographer: Fan Ruiqi

Foreword

SARS-CoV-2 is a novel coronavirus that is featured by high infectivity and rapid spread. Transmission of SARS-CoV-2 occurs through droplets and can happen through close personal contact with infected persons. Coronavirus disease 2019 (COVID-19) caused by caused by SARS-CoV-2 has been identified and reported in China and many other countries since late 2019.

As huge number of patients overwhelmed the admission capacity of infectious diseases hospitals in Wuhan, Hubei Province, Zall Foundation proposed the construction of COVID-19 Emergency Hospitals to admit the surging number of COVID-19 cases. Emergency Hospitals involve the conversion of existing hospitals that currently do not have, or have insufficient admission capacities for infectious disease patients, into emergency hospitals that solely focus on receiving suspected and confirmed COVID-19 cases. COVID-19 Emergency Hospitals have played a key role in China's epidemic prevention and control by efficiently offering the urgently required beds during the epidemic.

Based on the experience of constructing and operating these Emergency Hospitals in strict adherence to relevant medical standards and regulations, this booklet was compiled by the Zall Foundation crew who had participated in the rebuilding and supporting of Emergency hospitals, with an attempt to inform the ongoing renovations of Emergency Hospitals worldwide and thus contribute to the glabal efforts in combating the COVID-19 pandemic

Yan Zhi

Founder, Zall Foundation

April 2020

Contents

Chapter I   Background of COVID-19 Emergency Hospitals Construction

1.1   Background

Infectious diseases are caused by pathogenic microorganisms and can be spread, directly or indirectly, from one person to another. Among various types of infectious diseases, respiratory infectious diseases have the highest infectious prevalence rates and impose the greatest threat to the people's health.

The treatment of infectious diseases has higher requirements on medical environments and protective measurements. The patients can be only treated in a professional infectious diseases hospital, in order to prevent further cross-infection between patients and medical staff and so as to decrease the risks of disease outbreak. With the rapid development of medical technology and improved public health management, most infectious diseases have been contained and brought under full control, which results in the small number of professional infectious disease hospitals; on the other hand, the relevant medical supplies and resources would not be sufficient once an epidemic or pandemic occurs. In early 2020, coronavirus disease 2019 (COVID-19) rapidly spreads worldwide, resulting in inadequate and insufficient medical resources and supplies, which lead to the proposal on the Emergency Hospitals construction.

During the COVID-19 epidemic in Wuhan, Hubei Province, high patient numbers were overwhelming the admission capacity of designated infectious disease hospitals, leading to insufficient medical supplies fulfilling the treatment needs. In response to the surging number of COVID-19 cases, Zall Foundation proposed the "COVID-19 Emergency Hospital" construction plan. Along with seven professional medical institutions, Zall Foundation suggested converting these seven hospitals with no admission capacity for infectious disease patients into emergency hospitals that solely focused on receiving suspected and confirmed COVID-19 patients, which minimize the time and monetary costs. These seven hospitals included: the Eighth Hospital of Wuhan, Wuhan Hanyang Hospital, Huanggang Central Hospital Dabie Mountain Regional Medical Center, Wuhan Huangpi People's Hospital Panlongcheng Branch, Luotian No.2 People's Hospital, Jianli People's Hospital, and Suizhou Central Hospital. The renovations of these COVID-19 Emergency Hospitalswere completed within 2-5 days, and 4,583 wards in total were provided where 2,833 confirmed and suspected patients in Wuhan, Huanggang, Suizhou, and Jingzhou were cured.

Thus, COVID-19 Emergency Hospitals were established in the context of epidemic focusing on the treatment of suspected and confirmed COVID-19 cases. By converting existing professional medical institutions into designated hospitals, it addressed the problems of insufficient medical supplies and inadequate admission-capacities and played an important role in providing medical treatment and support.

1.2   Definition of COVID-19 Emergency Hospitals

The basic idea of Emergency Hospitals is to convert existing hospitals that currently do not have, or have insufficient admission capacities for infectious disease patients, into emergency hospitals that solely focus on receiving suspected and confirmed COVID-19 cases. After the renovation, the treatment environment, equipment and facilities, and operational management of these designated hospitals will have the same standard as a professional infectious disease hospital. The purpose of the establishment of the Emergency Hospitals is to provide patients with suspected or confirmed COVID-19 with medical care and frequent monitoring. The source of SARS-CoV-2 infection can also be isolated, which remarkably increases the recovery rate and decreases the infection rate. The reconstruction of existing hospitals involves lowest monetary and time cost and thus can rapidly expand the admission capacity and medical supplies.

1.3   The Function of COVID-19 Emergency Hospitals

(1) Screening and triage

A fever clinic is set up in the Emergency Hospital to

screen patients with laboratory tests, imaging examinations, and epidemiological investigations. This will help doctors to distinguish patients with common fever from suspected or confirmed COVID-19 patients. Patients will be triaged or admitted accordingly.

(2) Isolated observation and treatment of suspected patients

Before nucleic acid testing (NAT), all suspected patients from fever clinic should be observed separately. This will effectively lower the risk of transmitting virus to healthy people or being infected by confirmed patients.

(3) The admission and referral of confirmed patients

Confirmed patients should be provided with immediate medical treatment in isolated wards until they meet the discharge criteria. For severe and critical patients with worsening condition, they should be transferred to higher-level designated hospitals for COVID-19 patients.

Chapter II   COVID-19 Emergency Hospitals Project Design

The design of COVID-19 Emergency Hospitals should strictly comply with relevant regulation and standards including *Construction Codes on Hospitals for Infectious Diseases Control* (GB 50849-2015) and *Construction Standards and Regulations on Hospitals for Infectious Diseases Control* (Standard 173-2016).

2.1 COVID-19 Emergency Hospitals Project Design

(1) The signage system with functions including guidance and management should be implemented in COVID-19 Emergency Hospitals.

(2) All areas in COVID-19 Emergency Hospitals should be barrier-free and accessible.

(3) Hospitals should be strictly divided into restricted areas and isolated areas, where barriers gates should be placed in between. Logistics support facilities and essential living engagement supplies should be placed in restricted areas, whereas receptions, paramedical

rooms, wards, ventilation system, medical waste disposal facilities, temporary morgue, sewage treatment station and other medical support facilities should be placed in isolated areas. Restricted areas should be located in the upwind direction of isolated areas.

(4) Layout plan should comply with the principle of "three zones and two passages". Three zones are namely: contaminated zone, semi contaminated zone (potentially contaminated zone) and clean zone.

Clean zone: for medical staff who have low risk of exposure to patients' blood, body fluid, pathogenic microorganisms and other contaminated or infected materials. Confirmed patients with infectious disease are prohibited from entering the area.

Semi-contaminated zone: located between contaminated zone and clean zone, for medical staff who have medium-risk of exposure to patients' blood, body fluids, pathogenic microorganisms, and other contaminated or infected materials.

Contaminated zone: where confirmed and suspected patients with infectious disease are being treated and cured in this area. Blood, body fluid, secretion, medical waste and any contaminated materials are being disposed of in this area.

Furthermore, an operation workflow chart should be clearly informed and explained to all medical staff involved. The design of workflow should be unidirectional from clean zone to contaminated zone. There should be a buffer room between different areas, with wash basins and dirt buckets for polluted medical waste and surgery gowns. This will decrease the risk of cross-infection among medical staff.

"Two passages" are namely health workers passage and patient passage. Moreover, cleansing passages and contaminants transferring passages should be strictly separated to avoid any unnecessary interaction between medical staff and patients. The entrance and exit of the health workers passage should be located at the end of the clean zone, while the entrance and exit of the patient passage should be located at the end of the contaminated area.

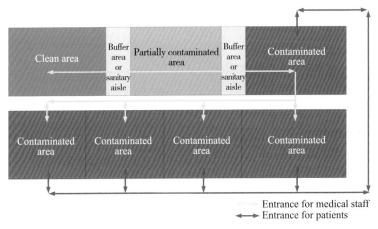

Fig.2-1   "Three Zones and Two Passages" Design

(5) The layout of the main medical building shall allow for the safe, convenient, reasonable, and efficient functional linkage among the clinical reception, medical laboratory, inpatients, and other main departments, which enhance the effectiveness of operation and management.

(6) Distance between buildings should satisfy the need of epidemic prevention and control. Distance between restricted area and isolated area should be no less than 30m. The distance between

buildings inside the isolated area should be no less than 20m.

(7) Complying with the hospital scale, there should be at least two entrances and exits. They should not be adjacent to main streets. The ambulance decontamination site and facilities should be set near the entrance and exit of the ambulance.

(8) Sewage treatment plant should be located at the low lying ground. The sewage should be easily discharged to urban drainage pipe after strict disinfection procedure

2.2　Reception Area Design

(1) The reception area should be located near the main entrance and exit.

(2) A clear clinical guidance for incoming patients should be placed at the entrance to avoid the overcrowding and cross infection.

(3) The entrance and exist of admission reception should be placed with buffer rooms.

(4) The consulting rooms, observation rooms, X-ray rooms, B ultrasound rooms, ECG rooms, treatment (preparation) rooms, dispensing rooms, temporary contaminant storage room, disinfection rooms, sanitary ware room, on-call room, doctor's offices, and toilets for medical staff should be set up.

(5) Patients can only access the consulting rooms, X-ray rooms, ultrasound rooms, and ECG rooms with the patient passage under the guidance of medical staff. All other facilities can be only accessed from medical staff passage.

(6) There should be a patient passage that directly links the

admission reception and ward area. This decreases the risk of further disease transmission.

2.3 Ward Area Design

(1) The wards with negative pressure and ICU should be provided for critical and severe patients, or "super spreaders".

(2) There should be a multidisciplinary consulting room and a telemedicine room if condition allows.

(3) Division of inpatient areas should be based on the disease conditions: suspected patients should be assigned to the single bed ward; confirmed patients should be assigned to the single bed ward or multi-bed ward; and severe patients, critical patients and "super spreaders" should be treated in the wards with negative pressure or ICU.

(4) Every inpatient area should be complemented with nurse stations, treatment rooms, disposal rooms, doctor's offices, on-call rooms, disinfection rooms, cleansing rooms, PPE storage areas, food preparation rooms, and boiler rooms.

2.4 Inpatient Room Design

(1) The beds should be parallel with the wall with clear glass. There should be 1–2 beds in a single ward (1 bed is preferred).

(2) For the ward with multiple beds, the passages between beds should be no less than 1.1m. The distance between wall and bed should be no less than 0.8m.

(3) Corridor in the single bed ward should be no less than 1.1m in width.

(4) The toilet in every ward should be complemented with a closet, shower equipment, and basins.

(5) The door of the patient room should be directly open to the corridor.

(6) Resuscitation room should be near the nursing station.

(7) Patient room door should be no less than 1.1m in width. An observation window should be placed on every door.

(8) Ventilation of the room should be in good condition. Patients can access fresh air outside through the window. Otherwise, an exhaust fan and ventilation system should be installed in the ward.

(9) Rail and anti-collision facilities should be placed on walls in corridors.

(10) There should be observation windows and delivery windows placed in between wards and medical staff corridors. Passthrough chambers should be used on delivery windows.

2.5 Medical Laboratory Design

(1) The patients waiting areas and the medical staff diagnose offices must be separated. There should be buffer rooms between medical staff working areas.

(2) Centralized drug warehouse and pharmacies should be located in clean zones, while daily-use medicine and equipment should be allocated in semi-contaminated zones.

2.6   Electrical and Intelligent Management Design

(1) Power system in the ward with negative pressure should be isolated and separated from others. Strong and weak electrical circuits and sockets should be properly sealed. Lighting and illumination control in the ward with negative pressure should be able to control in both ward and clean zone.

(2) Electrical circuits in different areas should be separately installed according to the division of clean, semi-contaminated, and contaminated zones. Major electrical installation should be located in the clean zone.

(3) Ceiling lamps in the ward with negative pressure should be properly sealed. During installation, any gap should be properly sealed as well. Materials of lamp shade should not be fragile, but with high transparency. The surface of the shade should be plain and easy to clean and disinfect.

(4) UV sterilizers and germicidal lamps should be installed in clean zone passages, filth cleaning rooms, toilets, inpatient rooms, waiting areas, treatment rooms, wards, and operating rooms. A device should be complemented with UV sterilizer in order to prevent any wrongful action. Switches should be placed at least 1.8m above the ground.

2.7   Water Supply and Drainage Design

(1) Draining pipe and ventilation pipe should be separately

installed for contaminated zone, semi-contaminated zones, and clean zones. Pipes should be made in corrosion protection materials.

(2) The valves of main pipes and branches of water supply should be located in clean or semi-contaminated zones.

(3) All hygiene equipment and floor drain should be complemented with water seals. Water seal should be no less than 50mm in diameter. Non-frequently used drains should be properly sealed.

(4) Rainwater of infectious area should be collected in the reservoir and go through a strict disinfection process before distributing to urban sewerage and drainage pipes.

(5) Contaminated liquid from hospitals should be centralized collected. After disinfection, it should be transferred into a septic tank and then distributed into the liquid disposal station. Contaminated liquid in the disposal station should go through a secondary biochemical process before being distributed into urban sewerage and drainage pipes.

2.8 Ventilation and Air Conditioning Design

(1) Mechanical air supply and air exhaust systems should be installed in the Emergency Hospitals. Air should be supplied and exhausted through pipes. The systems for different areas should be installed separately for clean zones, semi-contaminated zones, and contaminated zones.

(2) The minimum air exchange rate should be 12 times per hour in the negative pressure ward, 6 times in the semi-contaminated and

contaminated zones, and 3 times for clean zones.

(3) The condensed water from air conditioners should be collected in a centralized manner. It should be first transferred into the disinfection tank and then distributed into liquid disposal stations.

(4) In case the air conditioners are used in wards, packaged terminal air conditioners should be able to work independently. If any terminal is found to be simultaneously serving two more wards, the air condition should be immediately turned off, and replaced with a VRF system.

(5) The negative pressure difference controlled by the exhaust fans and ventilation system should be at the highest in clean zones, lowest in contaminated zones. The pressure difference between isolated wards and corridors should be at least 5Pa. Micromanometer should be installed on the wall of the clean area's corridor walls.

(6) Up-supply and up-exhaust air distribution schemes should be adopted in clean areas and semi-polluted areas. Up-supply and down exhaust air distribution schemes should be adopted in isolation wards. Air supply outlet should be located on the top of the bed-end, while air exhaust outlet should be located on the top of the head of the bed.

(7) The exhaust fans and ventilation system in the negative pressure ward should be working independently. Filter devices should be complemented with pressure gauges and safety alarms. Ventilation system should not be serving more than 6 words simultaneously.

(8) Air supplied to wards should go through low efficiency, medium efficiency, sub-high efficiency filters in order. Air should go through a high efficiency filter before exhausting. The filter should be placed beside the air exhaust outlet.

(9) The air exhaust outlet-in the isolation wards should be placed at least 3m above the ground, away from the supply outlet, doors and entrance for at least 20m in a downwind direction. The location of the ventilation machine should ensure the negative pressure difference in the ventilation pipes is maintained. The exhaust fans and ventilation system should be controlled in order: Turn on the exhaust fan before the ventilation system; turn off the exhaust fan first and then the ventilation system.

Chapter Ⅲ   COVID-19 Emergency Hospitals Reconstruction

3.1   Reconstruction Procedure

Reconstruction of professional medical institutions into COVID-19 Emergency Hospitals involves steps shown (Fig.3-1).

(1) Referral of non-COVID-19 patients

To avoid the infection to the existing non-COVID-19 inpatients in the hospital, some patients should be transferred to other hospitals or discharged before the reconstruction takes place.

(2) Evaluation of the current hospital conditions and analysis of the reconstruction procedure

The current conditions of the hospital shall be evaluated in terms of hospital environment, ward area layout, patient room design, water supply, drainage system and other factors. The procedure should be further modified and improvised based on the construction standards of emergency hospitals for COVID-19.

(3) Reconstruction project design

The above evaluation and analysis results are being considered when designing the construction schemes for hospital renovation.

(4) Construction

The preparation of materials and equipment should consider the needs and requirements of the reconstruction process.

(5) Project delivery and operation

After the reconstruction, the project should be evaluated and inspected comprehensively. If all relevant criteria and standards are met, the hospital shall be delivered for operation and start to receive and treat COVID-19 patients.

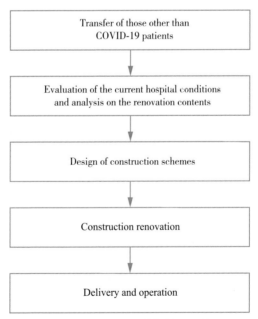

Fig.3-1　Reconstruction Process of COVID-19 Emergency Hospital

3.2   Reconstruction Project Design

The existing hospitals and facilities are partially reconstructed into temporary emergency hospitals for COVID-19 patients in the shortest time. It is the most realistic and accessible way to increase the medical resources and supplies for controlling the epidemic, and to improve the admission capacity for COVID-19 patients. The reconstruction project plan should strictly follow the project design of Emergency Hospitals in Chapter 2.

3.2.1   Reconstruction of Hospitals' Environment

(1) Hospitals should be strictly divided into contaminated zones, semi-contaminated zones and clean zones. An operation workflow chart should be clearly informed and explained to all medical staff involved. There should be a buffer room in between different areas, with a separate basket for the contaminated medical and surgery suits.

(2) Medical staff passages and patients' passages should be separately designed. Moreover, cleansing passages and contaminants passages should be strictly separated to avoid any unnecessary interaction between medical staff and patients. The entrance and exit of the medical staff passage should be located at the end of the clean zone, while the entrance and exit of the patient passage should be located at the end of the contaminated zone.

(3) Set up a special passage for the prevention and control of infectious diseases in existing hospitals, with prevention/containment facilities.

(4) The facilities and vehicles which are not involved in the

epidemic prevention and control around the Emergency Hospitals should be evacuated. For the nearby buildings which are located within 20m from Emergency Hospitals, necessary isolation measures should be taken (suspended the use of the buildings if needed). Citizens living around should be properly informed by signs and announcements.

(5) Indicate the location for the loading/unloading of medical supplies and equipment, and temporary storage space for epidemic prevention and control purposes.

(6) Indicate the ambulance cleaning and disinfection areas.

(7) Further environmental safety and protection measures should be taken for the medical waste and sewage disposal stations.

3.2.2   Reception Area Reconstruction

(1) Set up a fever clinic at the entrance of the hospital.

(2) Overall arrangement to the reception area should stick to the principle of "three zones and two passages".

(3) Mark out the screening area at the outpatient entrance.

(4) Make sure the reception area is provided with consultation rooms, observation room, X-ray room, ultrasound room, ECG room, treatment (preparation) room, sewage storage room, disinfection room, tool cleaning room, on-call room, locker room, doctor's office, doctor's washroom, etc.

(5) Patients can only access to the observation room, X-ray room, ultrasound room, ECG room, and entering from the patient passage under the guidance of medical staff. All other facilities can be only accessed and entered from the medical staff passage.

(6) There should be a patient passage that directly links to the

admission reception and ward area.

3.2.3 Ward Area Reconstruction

(1) Make overall arrangement to the ward area following the principle of "three zones and two passages".

(2) The negative pressure wards and ICU should be provided for critical and severe patients, or "super spreaders".

(3) There should be a multidisciplinary consulting room and a telemedicine room.

(4) Inpatient areas should be separately divided for suspected patients, confirmed patients with mild symptoms, and severe patients.

(5) Make sure the working area of each wards provided with nurse stations, treatment rooms, disposal rooms, doctor's offices, nurse's offices, on-call room, disinfection rooms, filth cleaning rooms, bedding and clothing warehouse, diet preparation room for patients, boiler room, and others.

3.2.4 Renovation of Normal Isolation Wards

(1) In the multi-bed ward, the distance between two parallel beds should be no less than 1.10m, and the distance between the bed and the wall should be no less than 0.80m.

(2) Corridor in the single bed ward should be no less than 1.1m in width.

(3) The wards shall be equipped with oxygen delivery, suction and other bedside treatment facilities, as well as call and intercom facilities. Make sure that there is enough room at the bedside for X-ray machines and ventilators.

(4) There should be observation windows and delivery windows placed in between wards and medical staff passages. Passthrough chambers should be used on delivery windows.

3.2.5   Renovation of Negative Pressure Isolation Wards

The procedure to modify normal wards into negative pressure isolation wards is as shown below. See Fig.3-2.

(1) Each negative-pressure ward is equipped with a toilet. A buffer room should be set between the passage for medical staff and the ward, where a non-manual or touchless faucet wash basin is provided. Pass-through chambers should be used on delivery windows.

(2) The ventilation system should be prevented from short circuit conditions of air supply and exhaust. The location of the supply outlet shall allow the fresh air to first flow through the working area for medical staff, and then to the wards. The air supply outlet shall be located on the ceiling. The air outlets of wards, consulting rooms and other contaminated areas should be located on the lower part of the room. The bottom of the air outlet in the room shall be no less than 100mm above the ground.

(3) Each negative pressure isolation ward should be equipped with a supply ventilation system with an air volume of $1,500m^3/h$. The air supplied to wards should go through low efficiency, medium efficiency, sub-high efficiency filters in order. There should be two exhaust systems, with one equipped with high efficiency filters. The air exhaust shall be filtered by the HEPA filter and then discharged. The HEPA filter for exhaust shall be installed beside the exhaust outlet in the room. Sealed valves should be installed on the air supply and exhaust pipes in each negative pressure isolation ward. The

sensor systems are equipped to control the variable frequency fans, to ensure that 5-Pa negative pressure is maintained between the negative pressure ward, anteroom and corridor.

(4) The negative pressure isolation ward should be the special first level load. Different low-voltage busbars from the existing substation (distribution room and electrical shaft) provide power to the wards by two-way power system, with one way for the emergency section, and a pair of power distribution boxes is equipped appropriately in the ward for the power supply. Different low-voltage busbars from the existing substation (distribution room and electrical shaft) provide power to the wards by two-way power system, with one way for the emergency section. and a pair of power distribution boxes are equipped appropriately for the power supply to the ward ventilation system.

(5) The exhaust fans and ventilation system should be controlled in order:

(6) ELV intelligent system

① The existing weak current system (data port, TV port, medical staff intercom port, fire detector etc.) in the ward remains unchanged.

② A building equipment's monitoring system is implemented to the ward, which automatically controls the ventilation system and monitors the differential pressure in the contaminated and partially contaminated areas.

③ In the ward, an access control system is added to control the passages for medical staff and patients, as well as the transition between contaminated and clean zones in the negative pressure wards.

④ A video monitoring system is implemented to the ward, with two-way voice and video communication functions.

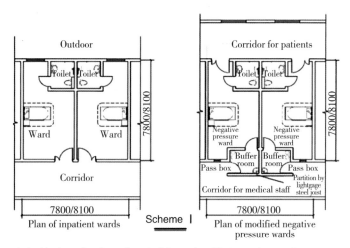

Note: A double-door closed pass box shall be equipped between the negative pressure ward and the corridor. A small buffer room is set between the ward and the corridor, and the doors are staggered to avoid the backfilling of air flow. The buffer room shall be provided with hand disinfectant, for healthcare workers to disinfect when getting in or out of the ward; besides, a waste pall is equipped to collect disposable wastes.

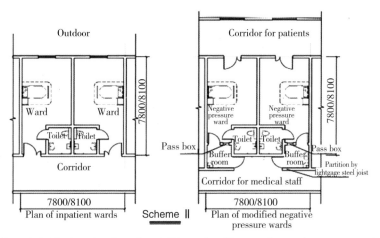

Note: A double-door closed pass box shall be equipped between the negative pressure ward and the corridor. A small buffer room is set between the ward and the corridor, and the doors are staggered to avoid the backfilling of air flow. The buffer room shall be provided with hand disinfectant, for healthcare workers to disinfect when getting in or out of the ward; besides, a waste pall is equipped to collect disposable wastes.

Fig.3-2　Renovation of Negative Pressure Ward in Emergency Hospital for COVID-19

3.2.6   Medical Laboratory Construction

Following the principle of "three zones and two passages", centralized areas of medicine and medical equipment should be located in clean zones, while daily-use medicine and equipment should be allocated in semi-contaminated zones. Consideration should be given on the separation of patients waiting areas and consulting areas. There should be buffer rooms placed between medical staff working areas.

3.2.7   Electrical and Intelligent Reconstruction

(1) Power system in the ward with negative pressure should be isolated and separated from others. Strong and weak electrical circuits and sockets should be properly sealed.

(2) The lighting fixtures in negative pressure isolation wards and clean rooms shall be clean and sealed, which is installed on the ceiling.

(3) UV sterilizers and germicidal lamps should be installed in-passage in clean zones, toilets, inpatient rooms, waiting areas, treatment rooms, wards, and operation rooms.

3.2.8   Water Supply and Drainage Reconstruction

(1) Draining pipe and ventilation pipe should be separately installed for contaminated zones, semi-contaminated zones and clean zones.

(2) The valves of main pipes and branches of water supply should be located in clean or semi-contaminated zones.

(3) Among the hygiene equipment, floor drain should be complemented with water seals, water seal should be no less than 50mm in diameter, and non-frequently used drains should be properly sealed.

(4) Floor drains in the consulting rooms, nurse rooms, treatment rooms, examination rooms, and washrooms isolated from the ward should be closed. There may be floor drains in the washroom of the ward, but regular inspection is required to replenish water for the water seal of floor drains.

(5) Make sure the outdoor sewage discharge inspection wells have closed manhole covers. The drainage pipe network is equipped with vent stacks, with the vent 2.0m above the ground.

3.2.9　HVAC Reconstruction

(1) Mechanical air supply and air exhaust systems should be installed in the Emergency Hospitals. Air should be supplied and exhausted through pipes. The systems for different areas should be installed separately for clean zones, semi-contaminated zones and contaminated areas.

(2) The minimum air exchange rate should be 12 times per hour for the negative-pressure ward, 6 for semi-polluted and polluted areas, and 3 for clean areas.

(3) The condensed water from air conditioners should be collected. It should be first transferred into the disinfection tank before being distributed into liquid disposal stations.

(4) In case the air conditioners are used in wards, packaged terminal air conditioners should be able to work independently. If any

terminal is discovered that simultaneously serves two more wards, the air condition should be immediately turned off and replaced with a VRF system.

(5) Make sure the isolation ward maintains a negative pressure difference of no less than 5Pa with its adjacent and connected buffer room and corridor. A micromanometer is installed on the wall of the buffer room in the clean area of each isolation ward.

(6) Up-supply and down-exhaust air distribution schemes should be adopted in isolation wards.

(7) Air supplied to wards should go through low efficiency, medium efficiency, sub-high efficiency filters in order. Air should go through a high efficiency filter before exhausting. The filter should be placed beside the air exhaust outlet.

(8) The air exhaust outlet should be placed at least 3m above the ground, and away from the supply outlet, doors and entrance for at least 20m in a downwind direction. The location of the ventilation machine should ensure the negative pressure difference in the ventilation pipes is maintained.

(9) Make sure the sewage drains and vent pipes in the ward areas are not connected to the drain and vent pipes in the non-ward areas. Good ventilation conditions around the vent pipe orifice of the upper roof shall be ensured, and gas disinfection facilities shall be provided at the vent pipe orifice if conditions permit.

3.3 Reference Cases of COVID-19 Emergency Hospitals for Admission of Diagnosed Patients

For the regions with critical epidemic situations and inadequate medical resources, where the confirmed patients cannot be sufficiently admitted, the renovated emergency hospitals for COVID-19 are solely used to admit the confirmed patients. This section introduces the renovation of the COVID-19 Emergency Hospitals for the admission of confirmed patients with Zall Changjiang Emergency Hospital (the Eighth Hospital of Wuhan) and Zall Hanjiang Emergency Hospital (Wuhan Hanyang Hospital) as examples.

3.3.1 Zall Changjiang Emergency Hospital

In order to alleviate the severe shortage of medical resources after the outbreak, Zall Foundation had worked with The Eighth Hospital of Wuhan to reconstruct the North Wing of the hospital. On January 30, 2020, Zall Changjiang Emergency Hospital was officially opened, which is also the first Zall Emergency Hospital for COVID-19. The Hospital has been equipped with a total of 300 beds, mainly for the admission of confirmed COVID-19 patients, and cumulatively treated 560 patients during its operation. The layout plans of the hospital renovation are shown in Fig.3-3 and Fig.3-4.

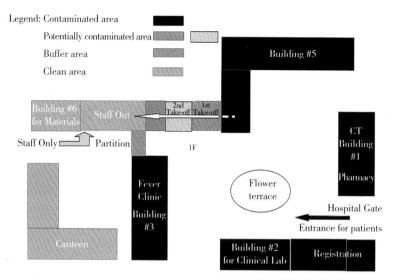

Fig.3-3   Layout Plan of Zall Changjiang Emergency Hospital 1F

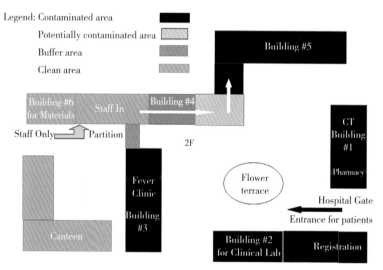

Fig.3-4   Layout Plan of Zall Changjiang Emergency Hospital 2F

3.3.2 Zall Hanjiang Emergency Hospital

On February 1, 2020, Zall Foundation worked together with Wuhan Hanyang Hospital in the renovation of Zall Hanjiang Emergency Hospital, which is solely focused on the confirmed COVID-19 patients. The general inpatient area was transformed into an isolation ward area in line with the standard of "three zones and two passages" within 3 days. After reconstruction, Zall Hanjiang Emergency Hospital increased its admission capacity to 260 beds and treated a total of 487 patients during its operation. See Fig.3-5, 3-6 and 3-7 for the renovation of the Hospital.

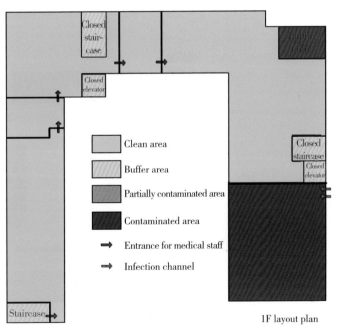

Fig.3-5 Construction Plan for Renovation of Internal Medicine Building 1F of Zall Hanjiang Emergency Hospital

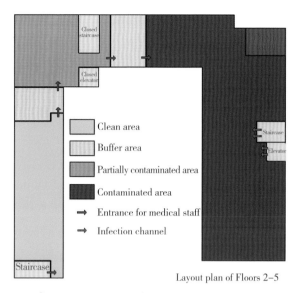

Layout plan of Floors 2–5

Fig.3-6   Construction Plan for Renovation of Internal Medicine Building 2-5F of Zall Hanjiang Emergency Hospital

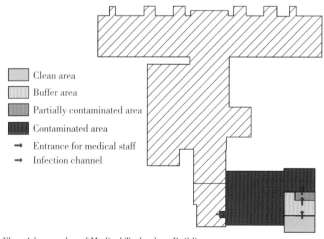

Floor 1 layout plan of Medical Technology Building

Fig.3-7   Construction Plan of Paramedical Building of Zall Hanjiang Emergency Hospital

3.4 Reference Cases of COVID-19 Emergency Hospitals for Admission of Suspected Patients

For the regions with less critical pandemic conditions and inadequate medical resources, where the confirmed patients are fully admitted but the suspected patients cannot be tested and treated, the Emergency Hospitals are developed mainly for the suspected patients. Taking Zall Panlongcheng Emergency Hospital (Panlongcheng Branch of Huangpi District People's Hospital), Zall Luotian Emergency Hospital (The Second People's Hospital of Luotian County) as examples, the following section introduces the reconstruction project of COVID-19 Emergency Hospitals for the admission of suspected patients.

3.4.1 Zall Panlongcheng Emergency Hospital

On February 7, 2020, Zall Foundation and Huangpi District People's Hospital worked together to renovation Zall Panlongcheng Emergency Hospital, renovated the inpatient wards of Internal Medicine and Pediatrics in Panlongcheng Branch of Huangpi District People's Hospital into isolation ward areas with "Three Zones and Two Passages" in line with the specification standards, and set up a total of 100 beds, solely used for the admission of suspected COVID-19 patients. During its operation, the Hospital has treated a total of 358 patients, and 123 patients have been cured. The layout plans of the hospital renovation are shown in Fig.3-8.

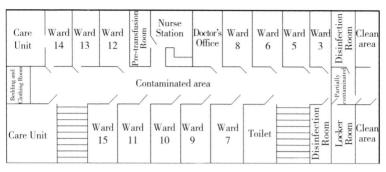

Fig.3-8   Layout Design for Isolation Wards of Zall Panlongcheng Emergency Hospital

3.4.2   Zall Luotian Emergency Hospital

On February 7, 2020, the Second People's Hospital of Luotian County and Zall Foundation jointly set up Zall Luotian Emergency Hospital. The Hospital has set up a total of 100 isolation wards totaling with 500 beds, mainly for the admission of suspected COVID-19 patients, and cumulatively received 192 patients, curing 180 during its operation. The layout plans for hospital renovation are shown in Fig.3-9 and Fig.3-10.

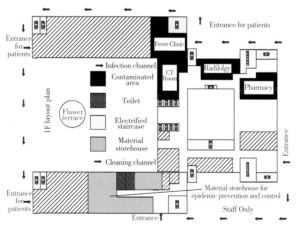

Fig.3-9   Layout Design of Zall Luotian Emergency Hospital 1F

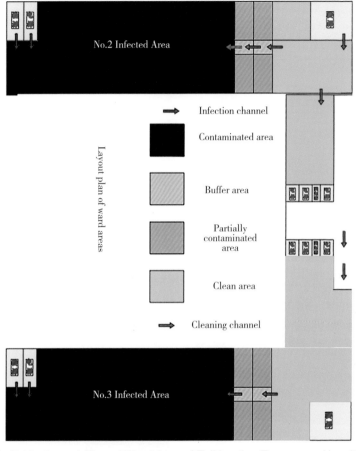

Fig.3-10 Layout Plan of Ward Area of Zall Luotian Emergency Hospital

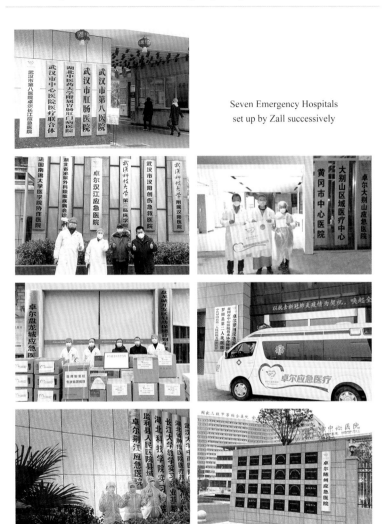

Seven Emergency Hospitals
set up by Zall successively

Fig.3-11 Zall Emergency Hospitals

Chapter Ⅳ   COVID-19 Emergency Hospitals Operation

4.1   Training Program for Medical Staff

4.1.1   Training Program Design

The training program is designed by specialists with extensive experience in teaching and epidemic prevention work from various clinical departments to ensure breadth of knowledge. The design of the program is in strict adherence to relevant medical standards and regulations, which will be tailored according to the actual situation of the hospital condition. The training courses and assessments mainly cover the procedures relating to proper hand hygiene, donning and doffing procedure of protective masks, gloves, goggles, face shields, protective suits and isolation gowns. Hierarchical protection, pre-examination and triage, as well as diagnosis, treatment and care should also be included.

4.1.2   Training for Medical Staff with Standardized Quality

Mentor team members will be selected from doctors and nurses of clinical skills training center. The training program for mentors consists of three stages. At the end of each stage, all selected mentors will be assigned into different groups, while the group leader is responsible for the evaluation of all trainee mentors, in order to ensure that standardized teaching quality has been delivered by the mentor team.

4.1.3 Scientific Design of Training Program

Based on clinical departments, experience level and professional fields, all existing medical staff shall be trained in order of expertise. To maximize the training efficiency, the program is divided into two parts: self-learning of theoretical materials and clinical operation training. Participants must complete theoretical self-study before participating in the onsite training. The onsite training procedure includes pre-class tests, watching teaching videos, detailed instructions given by mentors, practical simulation exercises and feedback given from the after-class assessment. During training, medical staff are able to directly apply the skills they have learnt to the practical operation.

4.1.4 Multi-Perspectives Evaluation

While the mentor team regularly evaluates the medical staff training performance from feedback collected, staff performance will also reflect the problems and inefficiency that appear in the training program. Attention also needs to be paid to suggestions and requests from medical trainees, which can be used to improve the teaching quality. See Fig.4-1.

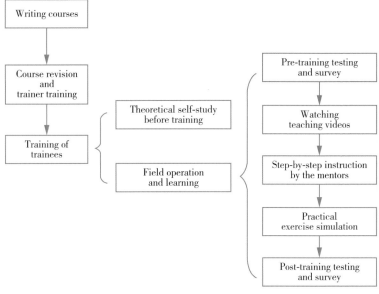

Fig.4-1   Training Procedure for Medical Staff

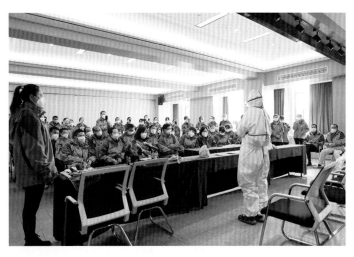

Fig.4-2   Pre-employment Training of Xi'an International Medical Center Hospital as Medical Team Invited to Aid Zall Changjiang Emergency Hospital in Wuhan

4.2 Patient Admission and Treatment

4.2.1 Pre-examination and Triage

The purpose of a scientific method of pre-examination and triage is to comprehensively monitor the condition of all patients and screen those at high risks of infection. Appropriate treatment in fever clinics in a timely manner will be provided to high-risk patients, which decreases the chance of cross-infection. The three-level triage system is shown below:

(1) Level-1 triage

Pre-examination and triage rooms shall be set up for patients with fever in the outpatient department. The infrared temperature thermometer is used to monitor the body temperatures of patients who enter the outpatient department. In case of any patients with fever (body temperature > 37.3℃) identified, they shall be re-measured with a mercury thermometer immediately. Meanwhile, their epidemiological information will be questioned. If the re-measured temperature is still higher than 37.3℃ , they must be accompanied by medical staff to the fever clinic for treatment regardless of their epidemiological information.

(2) Level-2 triage

Temperature monitoring points are set up at every nurse station in the outpatient department in order to monitor the body temperatures of all patients in a timely manner, and screen the patients with fever. Meanwhile, the epidemiological information will be collected from patients with fever. Patients with epidemiological evidence shall be sent to the fever clinic under the escort of a nurse. For patients without epidemiological evidence, they shall be guided to the fever clinic for further examination. After the possibility of COVID-19 is ruled out, they will be asked to return to the outpatient department.

(3) Level-3 triage

When diagnosing patients, the outpatient physician shall ask them whether they have a fever; if so, enquire about the epidemic medical history. For patients with epidemic history, the outpatient physician shall inform the nurses, who will accompany patients to the fever clinic; For patients without epidemiological evidence, they shall be guided to the fever clinic for further examination. After the possibility of COVID-19 is ruled out, they will be asked to return to the outpatient department.

4.2.2 Patient Admission Procedure

The physicians will first conduct laboratory inspection, imaging examination and epidemiological investigation to the patients in the fever clinic. The non-suspected patients will be generally treated and then asked to be home quarantined for observation, while the suspected patients are provided with treatment in isolated wards, with nucleic acid testing (NAT) which will be taken twice for at least 24hours interval. If the results are negative, the patients are given general treatment and then asked to be home quarantined for observation; if the NATs are positive, the patients shall be further evaluated by the symptoms and examination results. The patients with mild COVID-19 symptoms will be transferred to the Fangcang Shelter Hospital for treatment; the severe patients will be asked to be hospitalized for appropriate treatment in isolation. If patients fulfill the discharge criteria in the later stages, they will be transferred to the "Rehabilitation Station" (the isolation station for patients to receive rehabilitation treatment and medical observation) under quarantine observation and health monitoring for another 14 days.

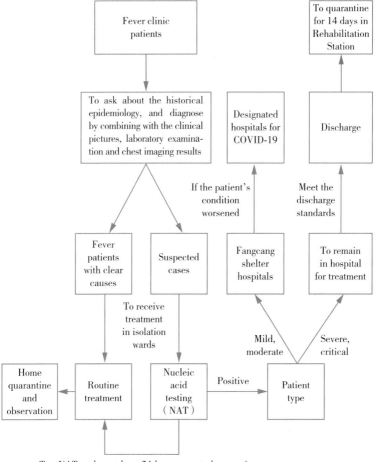

Fig.4-3   Workflow of Patient Reception/Admission

4.2.3 Patient diagnosis criteria

(1) Diagnostic criteria for suspected COVID-19 patients

With integrated analysis by combining the following epidemiological evidence and clinical symptoms, a patient would be defined as suspected case if one of the following is met: patient has any of the epidemiological characteristics along with any of two following clinical presentations or patient have all three clinical pictures if there is no clear historical epidemiology.

① Epidemiological evidences:

(a) History of travel to or residence in an affected area and its surrounding areas, or in other places where cases have been reported within 14 days prior to the morbidity.

(b) In contact with SARS-CoV-2 infector (with positive results for the nucleic acid testing) within 14 days prior to the morbidity.

(c) In contact with patients who have fever or respiratory symptoms from an affected area and its surrounding areas, or from places where cases have been reported within 14 days before the morbidity.

(d) Clustered cases (2 or more cases with fever and/or respiratory symptoms in a small area, such as families, offices, schools within 2 weeks).

② Clinical presentations:

(a) Fever and/or respiratory symptoms;

(b) The imaging characteristics of COVID-19;

(c) Normal or decreased WBC count, normal or decreased lymphocyte count in the early stage of onset.

If two NATs, taken in at least 24-hour interval, of a COVID-19 suspected case are negative, and the SARS-CoV-2 virus specific IgM and IgG antibodies are negative after 7 days from onset, the diagnosis of such suspected case can be ruled out.

(2) Diagnostic criteria for confirmed COVID-19 patient

Suspected cases can be diagnosed as confirmed cases if they have one of the following etiological or serological evidence:

① Real-time fluorescent RT-PCR indicates positive for SARS-CoV-2 nucleic acid;

② Viral gene sequence is highly homologous to known SARS-CoV-2;

③ SARS-CoV-2 specific IgM and IgG antibodies are detectable in serum; SARS-CoV-2 specific IgG antibody is detectable in serum or reaches a titration of at least 4-fold increase during convalescence compared with the acute phase.

(3) Clinical classification criteria for confirmed COVID-19 patients

① Mild cases. The clinical presentation and symptoms are mild, and there is no sign of pneumonia on imaging.

② Moderate cases. There are fever and respiratory symptoms, and pneumonia can be found on imaging.

③ Severe cases. Adult cases meeting any of the following criteria:

(a) Shortness of breath, RR $\geqslant$ 30 breaths/min;

(b) Oxygen saturation $\leqslant$ 93% at rest;

(c) Partial pressure of oxygen (PaO_2)/fraction of inspired oxygen (FiO_2) $\leqslant$ 300 mmHg (1 mmHg = 0.133 kPa).

In high-altitude areas (altitude > 1,000 meters), PaO_2/FiO_2 shall be corrected according to the following formula: $PaO_2/FiO_2 \times$ [Atmospheric pressure (mmHg) / 760].

Cases with chest imaging that shows obvious lesion progression (>50%) within 24 to 48 hours shall be managed as severe cases.

Child cases meeting any of the following criteria:

(a) Shortness of breath (< 2 months old, RR $\geqslant$ 60 breaths/min; 2 to 12 months old, RR $\geqslant$ 50 breaths/min; 1 to 5 years old, RR $\geqslant$ 40 breaths/min; > 5 years old, RR $\geqslant$ 30 breaths/min), excluding the effects of fever and crying;

(b) Oxygen saturation $\leqslant$ 92% at rest;

(c) Trouble breathing (moaning, nasal fluttering, and infrasternal, supraclavicular, and intercostal retraction), cyanosis, and intermittent apnea;

(d) Drowsiness and convulsions;

(e) Refusal to food or difficulty in feeding, and signs of dehydration.

④Critical cases. Critical cases must meet any of the following criteria:

(a) Respiratory failure occurs and mechanical ventilation is required;

(b) Shock;

(c) With other organ failure that requires ICU care.

4.2.4　Clinical Treatment for Patients

Suspected cases shall receive treatment in isolation in a single ward, confirmed cases can be admitted to the same ward, and critical cases shall be admitted to ICU as soon as possible.

The treatment and medical care provided for patients shall strictly comply with the newly issued *COVID-19 Diagnosis and Treatment Program*, *Nursing Standards for Severe and Critical COVID-19 Patients*, and *Treatment Guidelines for Severe and Critical COVID-19 Patients*.

4.2.5   Psychological Intervention Strategy for Patients

With such high patient numbers that are overwhelming the admission capacity, it is possible that patients will also generate negative feelings including depression and more. Hence, an appropriate level of psychological crisis intervention and sufficient mental health consultation for patients is essential, in order to make medical treatment more effective.

(1) Confirmed patients

① Newly isolated and treated patients

Patient mentality: numbness, denial, anger, fear, anxiety, depression, disappointment, complaining, insomnia or aggression, etc.

Intervention principles: focusing on giving mental support and showing empathy. Treat patients with patience, try to stabilize their emotions and assess the risk of suicide, self-injury, and violent acts in the early stage.

Intervention:

(a) Understanding that these emotional responses from patients are normal responses when facing intensive stress. Be mentally prepared in advance, showing professional care even when facing aggressive and negative acts from patients, for example, not quarrelling with the patient or getting excessively involved.

(b) Given the understanding of the mental status of patients, psychological crisis intervention shall be given in addition to medical treatment, such as assessing the risks of suicide, self-injury and violent acts in a timely manner, providing appropriate mental support, and avoiding having direct conflict with the patient. Patients can consult with a psychiatrist if necessary. Explain the importance of the isolation treatment to patients and encourage patients to build confidence towards future treatment.

(c) Emphasizing the purpose of isolation to the patients, explaining that it is not only for better observation and treatment, but also for the greater benefit of our family and community. Patients should be informed about the key characteristics of the treatment given and the effectiveness of any necessary intervention.

② Patients in isolation and treatment

Patient mentality: In addition to the possible emotional responses mentioned earlier, loneliness and fear of the disease may result in conflict rising with doctors, loss of faith in future treatments, or the opposite, namely unrealistically high expectations for the treatment.

Intervention principle: having direct communication more frequently with patients and providing essential information to stabilize their mental condition. Consult a psychiatrist if necessary.

Intervention:

(a) Based on patients' mental status, objectively and truthfully explain their health conditions, as well as the disease outbreak, so that patients are aware of the current situation.

(b) Encouraging patients to actively communicate with their families. Providing assistance if patients have any reasonable requests.

(c) Encouraging patients to cooperate with doctors in accepting any suggested treatment.

(d) Creating a comfortable environment with a soothing atmosphere that is suitable for patients' recovery.

(e) Having consultation with a psychiatrist if necessary.

③ Patients with respiratory distress, extreme restlessness, and difficulty in expressing themselves

Patient mentality: feelings of imminent death, panic, despair, etc.

Intervention principle: focusing on appeasing and calming the patients, paying attention to emotional communication with them, and helping them build confidence in treatment.

Intervention measures: While calming and appeasing the patient, strengthen the treatment towards the primary cause of mental issues and then relieve the stress.

(2) Patients with fever who seek medical care in the hospital

Patient mentality: panic, restlessness, loneliness, helplessness, being suppressed, depression, pessimism, anger, nervousness, stress of being distanced from others, grievance, shame, or disregard for the illness, etc.

Intervention principle: providing basic medicine education and encouraging patients to cooperate with any suggested treatment and adapt to rapidly changing situations.

Intervention:

(a) Assisting patients to understand the true and reliable information and knowledge from authoritative scientific and medical materials.

(b) Encouraging patients to cooperate with doctors in any suggested treatments and with any isolation measures. Ensuring essential living and social engagement needs such as a healthy diet and more.

(c) Help patients to build up confidence and have faith in future treatments.

(d) Patients are encouraged to seek social support to relieve stress by using modern communication methods to contact their friends, family, colleagues, etc.

(e) Encourage patients having consultation with psychologists using assistance hotlines or other online platforms to approach psychological interventions.

(3) Suspected patients

Patient mentality: hoping they do not have the disease, avoiding treatment, fear of being discriminated, or anxiety, asking for excessive treatment, frequent hospital transfer, etc.

Intervention principles: Give timely education and correct protection. Let patients understand the overall situation and obey instructions. Reduce their pressure.

Intervention:

(a) Receive education on relevant policies, conduct close observation, and seek early treatment.

(b) Adopt necessary protective measures.

(c) Comply with regulations, and report and explain any personal situation according to regulations.

(d) Follow mental health care guidance to relieve stress.

4.2.6   Discharge Criteria for Patients

Patients can be discharged if they meet all the following conditions. See Fig.4-4.

(1) The body temperature has been normal for more than 3 days;

(2) Respiratory symptoms have improved significantly;

(3) Pulmonary imaging shows a significant decrease of involvement in acute exudative lesions;

(4) Nucleic acid tests show negative twice consecutively on respiratory tract samples such as sputum and nasopharyngeal swabs (with sampling interval for at least 24 hours).

After the patient is discharged from the hospital, he/she shall be transferred to the "Rehabilitation Station" to receive the 14-day isolation management. Wear a mask to reduce close contact with others. Strengthen nutritional intake, drink plenty of water (more than 3000 ml per day), and gradually carry out indoor activities. Return to the hospital for follow-up and subsequent visits in two and four weeks after discharge.

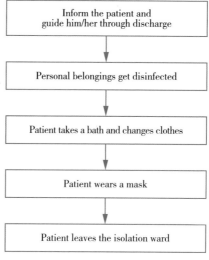

Fig.4-4   Workflow of Discharge

4.3   Medical Operational Management Policies

4.3.1   Management of Fever Clinics

(1) Operation and staffing: Fever clinics shall be opened 24/7 and managed by the emergency department. Trained physicians with clinical experience shall be assigned to screening, consultation, referral, and reporting of suspicious cases. In each fever clinic, there shall be two physicians simultaneously working, with two nurses providing assistance in the clean area. Furthermore, one more nurse shall be deployed in each fever clinic to coordinate work.

(2) Building layout: Divide the building according to the rule of "three zones and two passages" to ensure "unidirectional entry and exit".

(3) Frequent monitoring on ventilation system in the observation

room and resuscitation room; If mechanical ventilation is used, the air flow direction shall be controlled to flow from the clean side to the contaminated side.

(4) Medical staff shall be familiar with the epidemiological and clinical characteristics of SARS-CoV-2 infection symptoms, screening suspected patients according to the relevant diagnosis and treatment specifications, take immediate isolation measures for suspected or confirmed patients and report in a timely manner.

(5) Medical institutions shall provide masks for patients and accompanying personnel and guide them to wear the masks correctly.

4.3.2   Ward Management

(1) Suspected or confirmed patients shall be quarantined immediately and separately; suspected patients shall be isolated in single wards, and according to a etiological study, and confirmed patients can be placed in the same ward.

(2) Properly implement hand hygiene procedure and don/dof PPE when entering /leaving the isolation ward.

(3) Design procedures for medical staff's donning and doffing of the PPE; place a flowchart on the door and provide a full-body mirror. There shall be staff who are proficient in epidemic prevention and control work, to supervise medical staff's wearing and taking off PPE to prevent cross-infection.

(4) Stethoscopes, thermometers, sphygmomanometers and other medical equipment used for the diagnosis and treatment of suspected or confirmed patients should be used exclusively. If exclusive use of medical equipment cannot be guaranteed, it should be disinfected after use.

(5) Severe patients shall be admitted to the intensive care unit (ICU) or a ward equipped with conditions for monitoring and rescue. No other patients may be admitted to the intensive care unit (ICU) or the wards equipped with conditions for monitoring and rescue that are meant for admitting severe patients.

(6) Implement a strict patient-visiting system. In principle, no accompanying personnel is allowed. However, if the patient is under special situations and must be visited, the visitor must strictly comply with relevant regulations and containment measures.

(7) Intensify the ventilation of the ward, and sterilize the air with an air circulating disinfection machine twice per day.

(8) Sheets, quilt covers, and pillowcases used by confirmed patients shall be contained in double-layer medical waste bags, and the bags shall be labeled with "SARS-CoV-2 Infection" and sent to the starch washing and disinfection supply center for disinfection; Disinfect pillows, bedding, and mattress pads with a bed unit sterilizer. If there is visible blood or other body fluid contamination, treat it as infectious waste.

(9) General waste of patients with infectious diseases shall be treated as medical waste.

(10) Monitor the body temperature and symptoms of medical staff every day. If medical staff found with fever or respiratory symptoms, his/her health condition shall be immediately reported to the department of nosocomial infection management.

4.3.3 Patient Management

(1) Suspected or confirmed patients should be timely isolated,

and them should be escorted to enter the isolation area according to the specified procedure.

(2) Patients shall change into hospital gowns before entering the ward area. After patients' personal belongings and the changed clothes disinfected in a standard procedure, they shall be stored in the designated place and kept by the medical institution.

(3) Instruct patients to correctly choose masks and teach them the right procedure of donning the mask. Appropriate cough etiquette and hand hygiene should be educated.

(4) Strengthen the management of visiting personnel or accompanying personnel.

(5) For isolated patients, in principle, their movements are restricted to the isolation ward, which reduces the frequency of patient movement and ward change. If the patient really needs to leave the isolation ward or area, corresponding measures should be taken, such as wearing a surgical mask, to prevent the patient from causing contamination to other patients and the environment.

(6) When a suspected or confirmed patient is discharged from the hospital or transferred to another hospital, he/she can only leave after changing into clean and sanitized clothes. Medical staff are required to carry out disinfection of the all the facilities they have been in contact with.

(7) In case of the death of a suspected or confirmed patient, medical staff shall deal with the corpse in a timely manner. The treatment process is as follows: fill the corpse' mouth, nose, ears, anus and other open areas with cotton balls or gauzes that contain 3000 mg/L chlorine disinfectant or 0.5% peroxyacetic acid; wrap the

corpse with a double-layer cloth sheet, put it in a double-layer corpse bag, and send it to a designated place for cremation with a special vehicle. Personal items used by the patient during hospitalization can go with the patient or be taken home by his/her family members after disinfection.

4.3.4 Setup of ICU Ward Area and Human Resource Management in Nursing

(1) Setup of ward area

The setup of the ICU ward area shall be based on local conditions and reasonable layouts. It shall be strictly divided into the contaminated area, semi-contaminated area, and clean area. Set up a buffer area between the contaminated area, semi-contaminated contaminated area and clean area. Post clear signs in each area to prevent accidental entry. At the same time, set up entrances for medical staff and patients and make sure the two entrances are separate.

(2) Equipment and facilities

① First-aid items and medicines: equip the medical institution with a certain number of ambulances and first-aid medicines, oxygen tanks and supporting devices, ECG monitors, ECG machines, defibrillators, syringe pumps, infusion pumps, supplies for endotracheal intubation, portable vacuum extractors, noninvasive ventilators, hemofiltration apparatuses, ECMO and other devices.

② Disinfectant equipment: air disinfection machine, disinfection machine, air purifier, watering can, etc.

③ Gas and negative-pressure equipment: Prepare a wall oxygen system with sufficient pressure and compressed air.

④ Other facilities: refrigerators, treatment vehicle, wheelchairs, medical carts, etc.

(3) Allocation of nurses and scheduling principles

① Manage the nursing based on the patient-to-nurse ratio of 1:6. The recommended duration for each shift is 4 hours.

② Nurses should be enriched with ICU professional background, and show professional competence and due care.

③ Nurses should be in good health condition and able to undertake high-intensity work.

4.3.5   Transfer of Patients

(1) Transfer requirements

① The on-board medical equipment and facilities (including stretchers) placed in ambulances used to transfer patients, shall be used exclusively in the ambulance. The driver's cab shall be strictly isolated and separated from the carriage, and a special "contaminated" area for placing protection contaminants should be provided in the ambulance. The additional medical supplies include PPE, sanitizers, and disinfectants.

② Medical staff should wear full-sets of working suits, isolation gowns, gloves, medical cabs, and surgery masks. The driver must wear working suit, surgical mask, and gloves.

③ After the driver and medical staff transfer the patient infected with SARS-CoV-2, they must change into full-set of PPE in time.

④ Ambulances must be qualified for transferring patients with respiratory infectious diseases. When possible, use ambulances with negative pressure for transferring the patients. During transfer, the ambulance shall be kept in a hermetic condition. Disinfect the vehicle after using. When transferring severe patients, the vehicle should be equipped with the necessary life-supporting equipment to prevent the patient's condition from further deterioration.

⑤ The epidemic prevention of medical staff and drivers, the disinfection of vehicles, medical supplies and equipment, and the handling of contaminated items process and procedures should strictly comply with safety standards.

⑥ After ambulance returns, it needs to be disinfected inside-out before transferring the next patient.

(2) Transfer classification and configuration

The full-time chief resident or the second-line physician on duty determines the transfer level, to be transferred personnel and the items preparation based on the patient's pre-transfer situation and need for supporting means. According to the required supporting level of organ function, the transfer is classified into 5 levels: primary, intermediate, advanced, relatively contraindicated and absolutely contraindicated.

① Primary: For patients who only need to use a mask to inhale oxygen, use a low-dose vasopressor [dopamine $< 5\mu g/(kg \cdot min)$ or norepinephrine $< 0.1\mu g/(kg \cdot min)$]. The transfer personnel needs to include one doctor and one nurse from the related department.

② Intermediate: For patients who need mechanical ventilation, use a medium-dose vasopressor [dopamine: $5-10 \mu g/(kg \cdot min)$ or norepinephrine: $0.1-0.5 \mu g/(kg \cdot min)$]. The transfer personnel needs to include one physician from the ICU, one respiratory therapist (RT) and one nurse.

③ Advanced: For patients who need high mechanical ventilation support [oxygen concentration: 60% – 80%, PEEP: 10–12 cmH$_2$O (1cmH$_2$O $\approx$ 0.098 kPa)], use high-dose vasoactive drugs [dopamine: 10–15 µg/(kg · min) or norepinephrine: 0.5–1.0 µg/(kg · min)]. Patients are supported by ECMO. The transfer personnel needs to include one chief resident or second-line doctor from the department, one RT, and one nurse, or the ECMO transfer team.

④ Relatively contraindicated transfer: The patient's vital signs are extremely unstable or the internal environment is extremely disordered, and cardiac arrest will occur at any time and the patient needs to be rescued; The mechanical ventilation support required by the patient is very high (oxygen concentration $\geqslant$ 80%, PEEP $\geqslant$ 10 cmH$_2$O); The patient needs extra-large doses of vasoactive drugs [dopamine $\geqslant$ 15 µg/(kg · min) or norepinephrine $\geqslant$ 1 µg/(kg · min)]. It is suggested to rescue the patient on the spot and transfer the patient after the vital signs are slightly stable.

⑤ Absolutely contraindicated transfer: Medical staff are performing cardiopulmonary resuscitation on the patient, and after receiving cardiopulmonary resuscitation, the patient's respiratory status is still unstable under extremely high level of support (SpO$_2$< 90%, SBP < 90 mmHg).

(3) Transfer process

Wear protections$\rightarrow$ drive to the medical institution to pick up the patient $\rightarrow$ the patient put on a surgical mask $\rightarrow$ place the patient in the ambulance $\rightarrow$ transfer the patient to the receiving medical institution $\rightarrow$ disinfect the vehicle and equipment $\rightarrow$ transfer the next patient.

(4) Process of donning and doffing protective items

Process of donning protective items: wash or disinfect hands $\rightarrow$ wear a hat $\rightarrow$ wear a medical protective mask $\rightarrow$ wear a working suit $\rightarrow$ wear an isolation gown $\rightarrow$ wear gloves.

Process of doffing protective items: take off gloves $\rightarrow$ wash or disinfect hands $\rightarrow$ take off the isolation gown $\rightarrow$ wash or disinfect hands $\rightarrow$ take off the mask and hat $\rightarrow$ wash or disinfect hands.

Medical staff and drivers shall perform hand hygiene before going off work $\rightarrow$ shower and change clothes.

(5) Ambulance cleaning and disinfection

① Air: Open windows to ventilate.

② Carriage and object surfaces: Wipe and disinfect with hydrogen peroxide spray or chlorine disinfectant.

4.3.6　Protection Provided for Medical Staff

(1) Medical institutions and medical staff shall strengthen the implementation of standard preventive measures, manage the ventilation of the consultation rooms and ward area (patient rooms) well, wear surgical masks/medical protective masks, and wear disposal gloves when necessary.

(2) Take protective measures for droplet isolation, contact isolation and air isolation, and implement the following protective measures under different conditions.

① When contacting the patient's blood, body fluids, secretions, excretion, vomit and contaminated items: Wear clean gloves, and wash hands after taking off the gloves.

② When medical staff may be splashed by patients' blood, body fluids, secretions, etc.: Wear medical protective masks, goggles, and impervious isolation gowns.

③ When performing operations that may generate aerosols for suspected or confirmed patients (such as intubation, non-invasive ventilation, tracheotomy, cardiopulmonary resuscitation, manual ventilation before intubation, bronchoscopy, etc.):

(a) Take air isolation measures;

(b) Wear a medical protective mask, and conduct tightness test;

(c) Perform eye protection (for example, wear goggles or a face shield);

(d) Wear body fluid-proof long-sleeved isolation gowns and gloves;

(e) Carry out the operation in a well-ventilated room;

(f) Limit the number of people giving care and support in the room to the minimum needed by the patient.

(3) The PPE used by medical staff shall meet the relevant national standards.

(4) Surgical masks, medical protective masks, goggles, isolation gowns and other PPE shall be promptly replaced when they are contaminated with patients' blood, body fluids, secretions, etc.

(5) Use PPE correctly, wash hands before wearing gloves, and wash hands with running water immediately after taking off gloves or isolation gowns.

(a) Surgical mask: Surgical masks shall be worn correctly in the pre-examination and triage area, fever clinics and the entire hospital. Replace the surgical mask immediately when it is contaminated or wet.

(b) Medical protective mask: In principle, use medical protective masks in areas such as fever clinics, isolated observation wards (rooms), isolation wards (rooms) and isolated ICU (area); when collecting respiratory specimens and performing tracheal intubations, tracheotomy, noninvasive ventilation, sputum suction and other operations that may generate aerosols. A medical protective mask is generally replaced every 4 hours, and can be replaced at any time when it is contaminated or wet. For other areas and diagnosis and treatment in other areas, in principle, medical protective masks are not used.

(c) Latex examination gloves: Latex examination gloves shall be used in the pre-examination and triage area, fever clinics, isolated observation wards/patient rooms, isolation wards/patient rooms) and isolated ICUs. Put on and take off the gloves correctly and have the gloves be replaced in time. It is forbidden to leave the diagnosis and treatment area with gloves. Hand hygiene cannot be replaced by wearing gloves.

(d) Alcohol-based hand rub: medical staff shall use it when there is no obvious contaminant on the hands during the diagnosis and treatment. It shall be used throughout the hospital. The pre-examination and triage area, fever clinics, isolated observation wards/patient rooms, isolation wards/patient rooms and isolated ICUs must be equipped with the alcohol-based hand rub.

(e) Goggles: Use goggles in areas such as isolated observation wards/patient rooms, isolation wards/patient rooms and isolated ICU/patient rooms, and when collecting respiratory specimens, and performing tracheal intubations, tracheotomy, noninvasive ventilation, sputum suction and other operations that may generate splashes of blood, body fluids and secretions. It is forbidden to leave the above-mentioned area with goggles. If the goggles are reusable, they shall be disinfected before reuse. In principle, goggles are not used in other areas and for diagnosis and treatment in other areas.

(f) Protective masks/protective face shields: Use protective masks/protective face shields for the diagnosis and treatment that may generate splashes of blood, body fluids, secretions, etc. If it is reusable, it shall be disinfected before reuse; If it is for onetime use, it must not be reused. It is forbidden to leave the above-mentioned area with protective masks/protective face shields.

(g) Isolation gowns: Use isolation gowns in the pre-examination and triage area and fever clinics, and use impermeable disposable isolation gowns in isolated observation wards/patient rooms, isolation wards/patient rooms and isolated ICUs. For other departments or areas, use isolation gowns when in contact with patients. Disposable isolation gowns must not be reused. If the isolation gown is reusable, it shall be disinfected before reuse. It is forbidden to leave the abovementioned area with isolation gowns.

(h) Protective suits: Use protective suits in isolated observation wards/patient rooms, isolation wards/patient rooms and isolated ICU (area). Protective suits must not be reused. It is forbidden to leave the abovementioned area with medical protective masks and protective suits. In principle, protective suits are not used in other areas or for diagnosis and treatment in other areas.

4.3.7 Procedure of Donning and Doffing PPE

(1) Donning procedure of PPE for medical staff entering the isolation ward area and put on PPE

(Before entering the semi-contaminated area from the clean area)

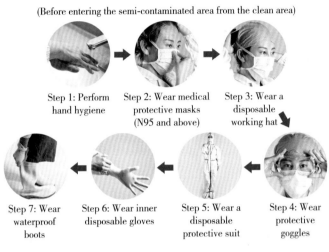

Step 1: Perform hand hygiene

Step 2: Wear medical protective masks (N95 and above)

Step 3: Wear a disposable working hat

Step 7: Wear waterproof boots

Step 6: Wear inner disposable gloves

Step 5: Wear a disposable protective suit

Step 4: Wear protective goggles

(Before entering the contaminated area from the semi-contaminated area)

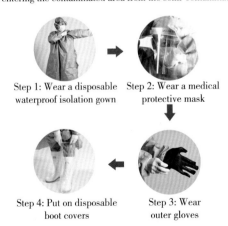

Step 1: Wear a disposable waterproof isolation gown

Step 2: Wear a medical protective mask

Step 4: Put on disposable boot covers

Step 3: Wear outer gloves

Fig.4-5   Procedure for Medical Staff Putting on PPE before Entering the Isolation Ward

(2) Doffing procedure of PPE for medical staff entering the isolation ward area

(Before returning to the semi-contaminated area from the contaminated area)

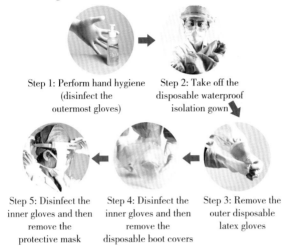

Step 1: Perform hand hygiene (disinfect the outermost gloves)

Step 2: Take off the disposable waterproof isolation gown

Step 5: Disinfect the inner gloves and then remove the protective mask

Step 4: Disinfect the inner gloves and then remove the disposable boot covers

Step 3: Remove the outer disposable latex gloves

(Before returning to the clean area from the semi-contaminated area)

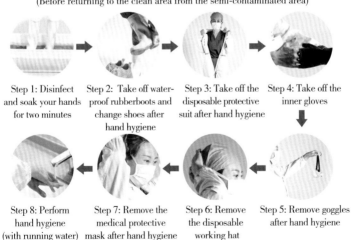

Step 1: Disinfect and soak your hands for two minutes

Step 2: Take off waterproof rubberboots and change shoes after hand hygiene

Step 3: Take off the disposable protective suit after hand hygiene

Step 4: Take off the inner gloves

Step 8: Perform hand hygiene (with running water)

Step 7: Remove the medical protective mask after hand hygiene

Step 6: Remove the disposable working hat

Step 5: Remove goggles after hand hygiene

Fig.4-6 Procedure for Medical Staff Removing PPE before Leaving the Isolation Ward

(3) Donning and doffing procedure of disposable surgical masks

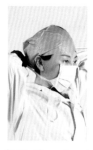 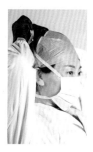 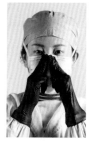 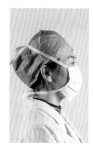

Step 1: The mask must cover the nose, mouth and chin, and the band under the mask shall be tied behind the neck.

Step 2: The upper band of the mask shall be tied to the middle of the head.

Step 3: Put your fingertips on the nose clip. Starting from the middle position, press inwards with your fingers, and gradually move to both sides to shape the nose clip according to the shape of your nose bridge.

Step 4: Adjust the tightness of the mask bands to fit your face.

Fig.4-7　Donning Procedure of Disposable Surgical Mask

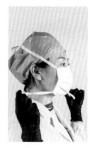 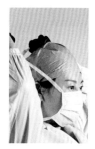 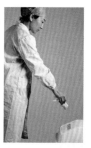 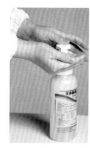

Step 1: First, untie the lower band without touching the front of the mask.

Step 2: Untie the upper band.

Step 3: Pinch the band with your hand and throw it into a medical waste bag.

Step 4: Perform hand hygiene.

Fig.4-8　Doffing Procedure of Disposable Surgical Mask

(4) Donning and doffing procedure of N95 respirators

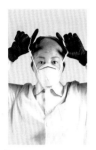 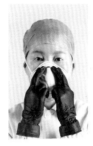 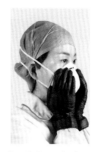 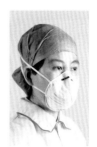

Step 1: The protective mask must cover the nose, mouth and chin, and the tip of the nose clip shall be close to the face. Pull the elastic band of the mask with both hands. Pull it up and over the top of the head, and put it behind the neck and in the middle of the head.

Step 2: Put your fingertips on the metal nose clip. Starting from the middle position, press the nose clip inward with your fingers, and move and press it to the side to shape it according to the shape of your nose bridge.

Step 3: Press the front of the mask with both hands and perform a positive pressure tightness test: Deeply exhale. If it is positive pressure, then there is no air leakage; If there is air leakage, adjust the mask position or tighten the band.

Step 4: Perform negative pressure tightness test: Inhale deeply. If there is no air leakage, the mask will be close to the face. If there is air leakage, adjust the mask position or tighten the band.

Fig.4-9   Donning Procedure of Medical Protective Mask

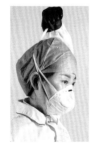 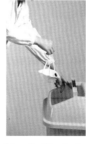 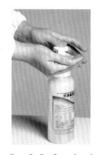

Step 1: Hold the two elastic bands with both hands at the same time, and lift them up and over the head to take the mask off.

Step 2: Pinch the elastic bands with both hands and throw the mask into a medical waste bag.

Step 3: Perform hand hygiene.

Fig.4-10   Doffing Procedure of Medical Protective Mask

(5) Donning and doffing procedure of isolation gown

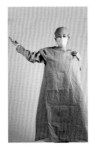

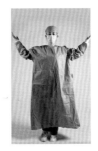

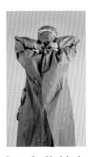

Step 1: Hold the collar with your left hand and put your right hand into the sleeve. Use your left hand to pull the collar upwards to let your right hand be exposed to the air.

Step 2: Now change sides. Hold the collar with your right hand and put your left hand into the sleeve. Let your right hand be exposed to the air. Do not touch your face.

Step 3: Hold the collar with both hands, and fasten the neckband backwards from the center of the collar and along the edge.

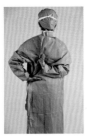

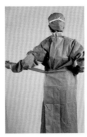

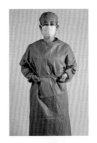

Step 4: Align the hem with your hands behind your back.

Step 5: Fold to one side, hold the fold with one hand, and pull the belt to the fold at the back with the other hand.

Step 6: Cross the ends of the belt behind, go back to the front, and fasten the ends of the belt.

Fig.4-11　Donning Procedure of Isolation Gown

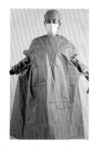

Step 1: Untie the belt and tie a slip knot in front.

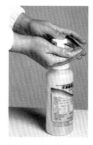

Step 2: Disinfect your hands.

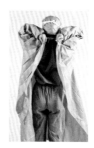

Step 3: Untie the band behind the neck.

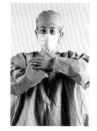

Step 4: Put your right hand into your left sleeve and pull the sleeve off your left hand.

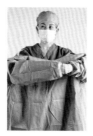

Step 5: Hold the outside of the right sleeve of the isolation gown with your left hand, which is covered by the left sleeve, and pull down the right sleeve.

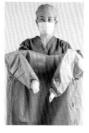

Step 6: Withdraw your hands gradually from the sleeves and take off your isolation gown.

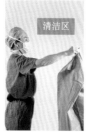

清洁区

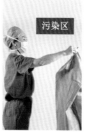

污染区

Step 7: Hold the collar with your left hand, and align the two sides of the isolation gown with your right hand. If you hang it in the contaminated area, the contaminated side of the isolation gown faces outwards. If you hand it outside the contaminated area, the contaminated side of the isolation gown faces inwards.

Step 8: When it is no longer in use, roll the used isolation gown into the shape of a package with its contaminated side facing inwards and throw it to the designated recycling place.

Fig.4-12   Doffing Procedure of Isolation Gown

(6) Donning and doffing procedure of protective suit

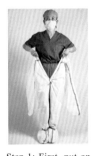 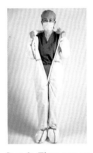 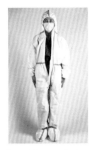 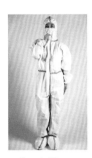

Step 1: First, put on the bottom.

Step 2: Then put on the upper clothes.

Step 3: Put on the hat.

Step 4: Zip up.

Fig.4-13   Donning procedure of isolation gown

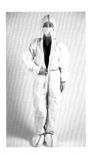 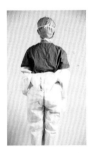 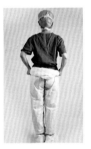

Step 1: Zip up from the top to the bottom.

Step 2: Take off the sleeves.

Step 3: Take off the protective suit from the top to the bottom and roll it with the contaminated side facing inwards at the same time. After rolling the suit into the shape of a package, throw it to a medical waste container.

Fig.4-14   Doffing Procedure of Protective-Suit

(7) Donning and doffing procedure of goggles or protective masks

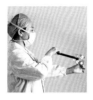

Step 1 : Check for any damage and slack.   Step 2 : Grasp the ear or head band of the goggles or protective mask and adjust it to make yourself comfortable.

Fig.4-15   Donning procedure of goggles or a protective mask

Step 1 : Grab the ear circumference of the goggles or the head and tail of the protective mask then remove the goggles.   Step 2 : For reusable items-Put in the container for centralized cleaning and disinfection. Non-reusable items-to discard into yellow medical waste bin, thereafter disinfect both hands.

Fig.4-16   Process of Taking Off Goggles or Protective Clothing Mask

4.3.8   Protective Supply Allocation

(1) Zoning based on exposure risk level

According to different exposure risk levels, medical staff workers who have resumed daily diagnosis and treatment will take on different personal protective measures.

① High risk exposure areas: All medical staff who directly or may come into contact with patients or their contaminants and the surfaces of the contaminated items and environment. The following departments are included: ICU, Emergency, the pre-examination and triage, fever clinics, emergency surgery, Clinical Laboratory, delivery room, catheter room, dialysis room and other departments in which invasive operations are performed.

②Low risk exposure areas: Personnel who are less likely to directly come into contact with patients or their contaminants and the surfaces of the contaminated items and environment. The following areas are included: General outpatient clinics, inpatient wards, Medical Laboratory, front-line managing staff and workers (cleaning staff, rotating warehouse staff, security staff, cafeteria staff, mortuary staff, medical waste disposal staff, accompanying staff, etc.).

(2) Allocation standard

In principle, allocate different medical protective supplies according to different risk exposure levels and different job requirements.

①High risk exposure areas

Items: Medical protective suit, medical protective mask, goggles or protective mask, isolation gown, disposable surgical mask, disposable working hat, disposable medical gloves.

Allocation standard: In the ICU, emergency surgery, clinical Laboratory, delivery room, catheter room, dialysis room and other departments in which invasive operations are performed, medical staff must be equipped with medical protective suits, medical protective masks, goggles or protective masks, disposable working hats, disposable medical gloves when diagnosing and treating all patients who are admitted by emergency department and haven't completed the COVID-19 screening.

②Low risk exposure areas

Items: Medical protective mask or surgical mask, disposable working cap, disposable medical gloves, working suit or isolation gown.

Allocation standard: All personnel in the medical institutions shall be equipped with those items.

Chapter V   Emergency Hospitals Logistics Support

5.1   Material Storage and Support

5.1.1   Storage of Common Supplies

(1) Common medicines

As for today, there is no known proven medicine or cure for COVID-19; however, the following drugs may mitigate the disease empirically:

① Alpha-interferon: 5 million IU or equivalent dose each time for adults, adding 2ml of sterilized water, atomization inhalation twice daily.

② Lopinavir / Ritonavir: 200mg/50mg per pill for adults, two pills each time, twice daily, no longer than 10 days.

③ Ribavirin: suggested to be used jointly with interferon or lopinavir/ritonavir, 500mg each time for adults, twice or three times of intravenous injection daily, no longer than 10 days.

④ Abidor: 200mg tid for adults, no longer than 10 days.

⑤ Chloroquine phosphate: 500 mg bid for adults, no longer than 10 days.

Apart from the drugs mentioned above, drugs such as antiviral drugs, antibacterial agents, analgesic-antipyretic, antitussives, antiasthmatic and expectorant medicine, gastrointestinal drugs, intestinal microecological modulators, and immunomodulators can also mitigate the disease. The hospital should reserve sufficient supplies of drugs according to admission capacity.

(2) Common device and equipment

Testing and monitoring equipment: Infrared thermometer, PCR detector, and patient monitor.

Therapeutic equipment: ventilators, oxygen machines, defibrillators, and injection pumps.

Disinfection equipment: temperature measurement and sterilization station and UV disinfection lamp.

(3) Common protective equipment

Operating caps, surgical masks, N95 respirators, working gowns, disposable coveralls, high-grade protective suits, full-face respirator masks, positive pressure headgears, goggles, disposable isolation gowns, protective shoe covers, and disinfectants.

5.1.2   Procurement and Supply

The hospital is responsible for tabulating the list of necessary drugs, protective equipment, and devices required, which will be subsequently purchased by the charity institutions. Other than ensuring common medical supplies mentioned in the earlier section, the hospital should also focus on ensuring adequate supply of drugs related to COVID-19 treatment. The purchase must be made from pharmaceutical companies with legal qualifications. The qualifications of relevant companies and business personnel must be recorded alongside the purchase for transparency and accountability. When there is a shortage of supplies, the hospital should actively negotiate and communicate with the providers, encouraging them to expand the supply chain or transfer the supplies from other regions. Meanwhile, if the purchasing process is difficult, the hospital should actively seek alternative supplies and materials.

5.1.3 Donation of Drug and Medicine

The donated drugs and medicines must meet the following requirements and criteria:

① For those produced within China, the drug must be a product approved by the national drug regulatory authority, with valid approval number, and meet quality standards. The validity period must be more than 6 months before the expiration.

② For those produced outside of China, the drug should be approved by the local drug regulatory authority, accepted by international pharmacopoeia, legally produced and listed in the country of registration, and meet quality standards. The validity period must be more than 6 months before the expiration. For approval that is valid for only 12 months, the drug must be valid for at least 6 months.

5.2   Warehouse and Logistics Support

To improve the efficiency of management and resource utilization, the medical and living materials and supplies are under unified management and storage systems. Meanwhile, a professional transport team is formed to allocate supplies in time according to the actual demand.

5.2.1   Warehouse Management System

(1) Responsibilities:

① Goods receiving, warehouse entry, returning, storage and protection.

② Loading and unloading, transportation and packaging of supplies.

③ Disposal of waste.

(2) Management Requirements:

① For each arriving shipment of supplies, before the supplies are stored into the warehouse, the go-down entry should be issued once the supplies are checked.

② According to the demand of supplies, after the consignor and the transportation vehicle have been checked correctly, the outbound order is made and signed by the consignor.

③ On a daily basis, the warehouse must make inventory tables and distribution charts for unallocated supplies, and keep the supplies classified and preserved properly.

5.2.2 Transportation Management System

Transportation agencies must follow a unified command and coordination plan. They must propose and formulate plausible transportation plans, and deliver the supplies and materials to COVID-19 Emergency Hospital in a safe and timely manner. See Fig 5-1 and Fig 5-2.

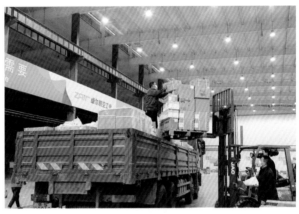

Fig.5-1　Warehouse of Zall Emergency Hospital

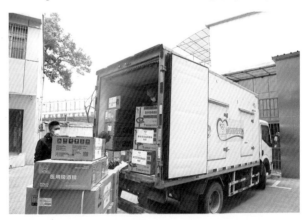

Fig.5-2　Allocation of Materials of Zall Emergency Hospital

5.3   Dietary Nutrition Support

5.3.1   Dietary Guidelines

(1) Diet plan for patients with mild symptoms and recovery patients

① In order to maintain adequate daily energy, patients should ensure sufficient nutritional intake, such as: daily intake of 250–400g cereal and tubers, which includes: rice, flour, grains and others; daily intake of 150–200g protein, which includes: lean meat, fish, shrimp, eggs, beans and more; consume one egg daily if it is possible, along with 300g of milk and dairy products (yogurt can be selected as it can provide essential probiotics). Moreover, it is important to ensure fatty-acid intake through various types of vegetable oil, especially through those with unsaturated fatty-acid. Total fat should reach 25% to 30% of total energy intake.

② Patients should be encouraged to eat more fresh fruits and vegetables: 500g daily vegetables intake and 200–350g daily fruits intake (dark green vegetables would be recommended).

③ Patients should drink enough water (1500–2000ml daily). Patients should drink boiled water or tea. Soup made from vegetables, fish or chicken is also recommended to be consumed drink before or after meals. Drinking water in small amounts, but more frequently can help increase water intake.

④ Eating wild animals is strictly prohibited. Food with spicy flavor is not recommended.

⑤ A special diet plan will be provided to patients with anorexia, chronic diseases and elderly patients, with nutrient intensifying supplements including: proteins, Vitamins A, B, C, D and other types of micronutrients.

(2) Diet plan for severe patients

It is common that severe patients often have decreasing appetite, which leads to insufficient energy and nutritional intake. This will lessen resistance to the disease. Hence, greater attention should be paid on the dietary plan for severe patients. The following principles should be followed when setting daily nutritional intake:

① Consuming smaller meals, but more frequently will help increase food intake. Consume liquid food 6 to 7 times a day (liquid diet is easier to swallow and digest). Patients are encouraged to eat more egg, beans, milk and dairy products, fruit juice, vegetable juice and rice flour. Good protein is also important for daily nutrition intake. During the recovery period, a semi-liquid diet can be taken. When the health condition is stable, a normal diet plan can be provided for patients.

② If food consumed by severe patients fails to meet daily nutrition intake standards, special medical-use food can be provided such as food containing enteral nutritional supplement, under the guidance of medical staff.

③ Under the circumstances of insufficient enteral nutrition, loss of intake ability, or facing a patient with severe gastrointestinal dysfunction, parenteral nutrition should be used in order to maintain basic nutrition daily intake. Parenteral nutrition should be 60% to 80% of total nutritional intake in the early stage, and increased to the full amount when patients' health condition is better.

④ Diet for severe patients should be planned based on body condition, intake and output volume, hepatorenal function, and glucose/lipid metabolism of the patients.

(3) Diet Plan for frontline medical support staff

A balanced diet plan for front-line medial and support staff should comply with the following principles:

① In order to ensure adequate daily energy intake, male staff are encouraged to consume 2400 – 2700 kcals a day, while female staff are encouraged to consume 2100 – 2300 kcals a day.

② Staff should ensure there is adequate daily consumption of protein, such as egg, milk, meat, fish and shrimp, beans and more.

③ Food with light texture is recommended, and greasy foods should be avoided. Natural spices can be used as ingredients to increase appetites.

④ Foods with enriched vitamin B and C, minerals and dietary fiber is encouraged, along with rice and noodles, vegetables and fruits. Black vegetables such as rape, spinach, celery, purple cabbage, carrot, tomato, orange, apples and kiwi fruits, as well as homonemeae vegetables such as mushrooms and seaweed are also recommended in daily diet.

⑤ Water intake should be 1500ml to 2000ml per day.

⑥ When a normal diet plan cannot meet the daily nutritional intake standard, enteral nutrition supplements can be used under the guidance of medical staff, together with powdered milk and other supplements. Additional 400kcals to 600kcals of oral nutrition supplements should be administered a day, in order to ensure daily energy intake.

⑦ Eating alone should be promoted, to effectively decrease the risk of cross-infection during meal times by avoiding gathering.

⑧ Departments which are responsible for diet plans should reasonably adjust measures in line with the conditions of the frontline medical and support staff.

5.3.2 Logistics and Distribution Management

The Emergency Hospitals' own logistics support teams have faced with difficulties in delivering sufficient amounts of food for patients and medical staff since COVID-19 outbreak. Meanwhile, the F&B industry is deeply affected by the epidemic, causing the closing down of restaurants. Facing such pressing conditions, charities and nonprofit organizations should collaborate with medical institutions, not only for the setting of diet plans, but also for finding suitable logistics and distribution companies to deliver essential food supplies. Taking Zall Hanjiang Emergency Hospital as an example, the logistics and distribution company delivers food to the quarantine building with refrigerated trucks, the hospital's logistics support crew then arranges for staff to pick up the food supplies, then deliver them to different cleaning areas according to the amount reported. Finally, food will be sent to wards by the nurses on duty.

5.4　Hygiene and Disinfection

5.4.1　Air Disinfection

Daily basis: At least 4 times a day. Disinfect the room immediately once after suspected or confirmed patients are treated.

Occupied room: Natural ventilation 30 minutes every time. UV air disinfection 2 hours every time.

Empty room: The disinfection method for "Occupied room" is applicable. Disinfection by lamp irradiation.

Final disinfection: Disinfectants such as peracetic acid, chlorine dioxide, hydrogen peroxide, etc. can be used for disinfection by using the ultralow volume spray method. After the disinfection, the room must be ventilated thoroughly.

5.4.2　Surface and Environment Disinfection

Disinfection on daily basis: 4 times every day

Disinfection on timely basis: After treating suspected or confirmed patients, the room and transfer devices must be disinfected.

Final disinfection: after daily work

Disinfection method: Wipe or spray the object surface with 1000mg/L chlorine-containing disinfectant. After 30 minutes, wipe the surface with clean water. Clean the floor with 1000mg/L chlorine-containing disinfectant, the duration of disinfection must be at least 30 minutes.

5.4.3 Floor and Wall Disinfection

Evenly spray and disinfect the surfaces of corridors, lavatory, toilets, waste disposal, medical waste storage rooms, and other spaces with 1000mg/L chlorine-containing disinfectant. The process must be at least 30 minutes each time and 4 times every day. Clean the floor with a 1000mg/L chlorine-containing disinfectant, and the duration of disinfection must be at least 30 minutes, 4 times every day.

5.4.4 Medical Equipment Disinfection

Disposable medical instruments and equipment shall be used as much as possible, and dispose the medical waste after use. For those reusable medical instruments and equipment, first being soaked in 2000mg/L chlorine-containing disinfectant for 30 minutes, and then sealed in a special container with mark of "COVID-19" for recycling. For disinfection supply centers, pressure steam sterilization is recommended. For devices that are not heat resistant, chemical disinfectant or low-temperature sterilization is preferred.

5.4.5 Disposal of Patients' Blood, Excretion, Secretion, Vomit

(1) A small amount of contaminants can be carefully removed by disposable absorbent materials (such as gauze and cleaning cloth) after dipping 5000–10000mg/L chlorine-containing disinfectant, or removed by disinfectant wipes/dry wipes with strong disinfection effect.

(2) A large amount of contaminants shall be completely covered with disinfectant powder or bleaching powder containing water-

absorbing components. Or they shall be completely covered with disposable water absorbing materials before applying sufficient 5000–10000mg/L chlorine-containing disinfectant on the water absorbing materials for more than 30 minutes. They can also be removed by disinfectant wipes/dry wipes with strong disinfection effect. These contaminants shall be carefully removed. Contact with contaminants shall be avoided during removal. The contaminants shall be treated as medical wastes in concentration. Patient's excretion, secretion and vomits shall be collected in a special container and soaked in 20000mg/L chlorine-containing disinfectant with the substance to medicine ratio of 1 : 2 for 2 hours.

(3) After the removal and disposal of the contaminant, the surface of the environment and objects should be disinfected. The container holding contaminants can be immersed in 5000mg/L chlorine-containing disinfectant for 30 minutes.

5.4.6　Miscellaneous

(1) Patients' cutlery, leftovers, vegetable residue should be disinfected.

(2) During morning care, change the sheets with disposable bed covers. Each bed should have one bed cover. The patients' clothes, sheets, duvet covers and pillowcases should be replaced immediately after contaminated. The bedside table, bed, chair and stool should be wiped and disinfected with disinfectant on a daily basis. After the discharge or the death of the patient, the bedcover of the patient must go through final disinfection.

(3) When collecting patients' clothing, quilts and other textiles,

aerosols shall be avoided. It is recommended to incinerate them as medical wastes in concentration; Textiles that need to be reused shall be soaked in 20000mg/L chlorine-containing disinfectant for 30 minutes before routine cleaning. They shall be collected in water-soluble packing bags as infectious textiles and delivered to a cleaning company for cleaning and disinfection. Expensive clothes can be disinfected by ethylene oxide.

5.5   Medical Waste Management

5.5.1   Classification and Collection of Medical Waste

(1) Define the range of classified collection. Waste produced by medical institutions or hospitals during the treatment of confirmed or suspected patients with COVID-19, including medical waste and household garbage, should be collected, classified and disposed in the same way as medical waste.

(2) Establish strict standards for packaging and containers. Warning signs must be attached to the surface of special packaging bags and sharps container for medical waste. Before disposing medical waste, careful inspection should be carried out to ensure the container is not damaged or leaking. Foot operated and covered barrels are preferred for waste collection. When the medical waste reaches 3/4 of the packaging bag or sharps container, it should be sealed effectively and tightly. Double-layer packaging bags should be used to contain medical waste, and gooseneck-type seals should be used for layered sealing.

(3) Collect waste safely. According to the type of medical waste, collect the waste in a timely manner, ensuring the safety of personnel and minimizing the risk of infection. When the surface of the packaging bag and sharps container is contaminated with infectious waste, a layer of packaging bag should be added. It is strictly forbidden to squeeze the bag when collecting disposable clothing, protective clothing and other items after use. Each packaging bag and sharps box should be attached with a label. The label should include the name of medical unit, department, date and type of waste, and mark specifically with "COVID-19".

(4) Process the waste from different zones. For those medical waste produced by confirmed or suspected patients with COVID-19 at fever clinic and wards before leaving the contaminated area, the surface of the packaging bag should be sprayed uniformly and disinfected with 1000mg/L of chlorine-containing disinfectant, or a layer of medical waste packaging bag should be added on the outside. The medical waste generated in the clean zone should be disposed of according to conventional medical waste.

(5) Handle pathogen samples carefully. High-risk waste such as pathogen-containing specimens and related preservation solutions in medical waste should be steam or chemically sterilized at the place of production, then collect and dispose of the waste in the same way as infectious medical waste.

5.5.2   Transportation and Collection of Medical Waste

(1) Management of safe transportation. Before transporting medical waste, the personnel should check whether the label and

the seal of the bag or sharps-container meet the requirements. While transporting the waste, the personnel should prevent damage to the packaging bags and sharps containers containing medical waste, avoid direct contact with medical waste, and avoid leakage and spread of medical waste. Clean and disinfect the transportation tools with 1000mg/L of chlorine-containing disinfectant after the daily transportation. When the transportation tool is contaminated with infectious medical waste, it should be disinfected immediately.

(2) Management of handover and storage. The temporary storage place for medical waste should be tightly closed and attended by hospital staff, and prevent irrelevant personnel from coming into contact with medical waste. Medical waste should be stored in a separate and temporary area, and handed over to the medical waste disposal unit for disposal as soon as possible. The floor of temporary storage places must be disinfected with 1000mg/L of chlorine-containing disinfectant twice a day. The medical department, transport personnel, temporary storage staff, and medical waste disposal unit transfer personnel should check and register while handing over the waste, and explain to each other that it originates from patients with pneumonia or suspected patients infected with new coronavirus so that extra caution can be taken.

5.5.3　Disposal of Medical Waste

Irrelevant articles and personal necessities shall not be placed or stored in incineration sites. During the incineration, the medical wastes shall be properly packaged; After incineration, relevant equipment, containers and sites shall be thoroughly cleaned and sterilized. Medical waste disposal equipment should be cleaned and sterilized before repair and maintenance. Sewage generated during the disposal of medical waste (including disinfection and cleaning for delivery vehicles, containers, temporary storage facilities, and disposal of sewage on the ground) should be discharged after being disinfected by centralized sewage treatment facilities.

5.6   Mental Health Care and Support

Healthcare workers often face heavy mental and physiological stresses caused by the risky and highly-intensive work, which may affect their work enthusiasm and performance. With such high patient volume that overwhelmed the admission capacity, it is possible that patients will prone to suffer from negative feelings including depression, etc. Hence, it is essential to establish mental health care policies and show our support for frontline healthcare workers. See Fig. 5-3.

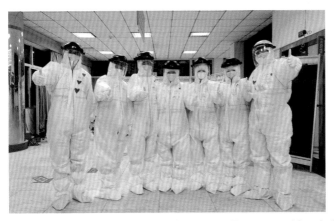

Fig.5-3   Group Photo of Medical Staff in an Emergency Hospital

5.6.1　Mental Health Care for Medical Staff

(1) Improving working and leisure facilities

Ensuring privacy by providing additional facilities such as single resting rooms for medical staff. Moreover, attention should be paid to the leisure and isolation needs, as well as essential living and social engagements of healthcare workers.

(2) Work and leisure balance

While providing medical treatment to patients, sufficient resting hours should be provided to medical staff, according to the current epidemic prevention and control conditions and relevant scientific research. Generally speaking, medical staff should not work consecutively over a month. Frontline medical staff should have a shorter consecutive working period. Deferred holidays leave should be arranged for those who are unable to take leave during the prevention and control working period, after they have completed their mission.

(3) Enhancing health care facilities for medical staff

Ensure sufficient medical supplies for containment, especially for staff working in the front-line. Physical examination should be given to front-line staff, including CT scans and more, which will decrease the risk of cross-infection. If any medical staff is found infected, immediate isolation and treatment should be provided.

(4) Psychological crisis intervention and mental health care consultation

A psychological consulting team should be established which consists of psychologists and other medical staff. Its major responsibility is to assess the health condition of every medical staff, while providing essential guidance. An appropriate level of psychological crisis intervention provided to medical staff and their families is also important, in order to effectively relieve the pressure they face. For medical staff having stress disorder symptoms, more mental intervention should be given, along with rearrangements of their working schedules to ensure adequate down time.

(5) Providing essential care to front-line staff

Understanding the needs and demands of front-line staff and their families, and fulfil reasonable requests from them in a timely manner.

(6) Human resource preferential policies

Based on the evaluation of medical staff's performance in epidemic prevention and control, additional credit should be given to outstanding medical staff. Preferential policies should be adopted by the medical institution's recruitment team; priority should be given to medical staff with outstanding performance in terms of promotion, title evaluation, etc.

(7) Welfare policies

Increasing salary and providing subsidies.

(8) Improving working conditions and ensuring safety at work

Strengthen safety measures and improve working conditions. No tolerance will be given to any direct or indirect discrimination to the medical staff and their families. Legal action will be taken towards tort, intentionally spreading of diseases and disorderly acts.

(9) Incentives

Give credit and commendation to medical staff who made significant contribution in the epidemic prevention and control and show outstanding performance.

5.6.2　Mental Health Care for Patients

(1) Psychological crisis intervention and mental health care consultation

A psychological consulting team should be established by psychologists and other medical staff. The major responsibility is to assess the health condition of every patient, while providing essential guidance. An appropriate level of psychological crisis intervention provided to patients is also important, in order to effectively relieve their pressure.

(2) Welfare and subsidies policies

Subsidies shall be granted for patients with financial difficulties, thus encouraging them to held positive attitude and cooperate with treatment.

References

[1] Ministry of Housing and Urban-Rural Development of the People's Republic of China. GB 50849-2014. Architectural Design Code for Infectious Diseases Hospital [S]. Beijing: China Planning Press, 2015.

[2] Ministry of Housing and Urban-Rural Development of the People's Republic of China. National Development and Reform Commission. Construction standards 173-2016 Construction Standard for Infectious Diseases Hospital [S]. Beijing: China Planning Press, 2016.

[3] China Association for Engineering Construction Standardization. The Design Standard of Infectious Disease Emergency Medical Facilities for COVID-19 [S]. Beijing: China Building Industry Press, 2020.

[4] Housing and Urban-Rural Development Department of Zhejiang Province. Health and Family Planning Commission of Zhejiang Province. Architectural Design Code for Infectious Diseases Area (Department) of Zhejiang Province [s. Hangzhou: Zhejiang Standard Design Station, 2006.

[5] Housing and Urban-Rural Development Department of Zhejiang Province. Technical Guide for Construction of Respiratory) Infectious Disease Emergency Hospital in Zhejiang Province (Trail)[Z.2020].

[6] Housing and Urban-Rural Development Department of Zhejiang Province. Technical Guide for Emergency Renovation of Deadly Infectious Diseases Area (Department) of Zhejiang Hospitals (Trail)[Z].2020.

[7] National Health Commission of the People's Republic of China Ministry of Housing and Urban-Rural Development of the People's Republic of China. Notice on issuing Design Guide for COVID-19 Emergency Facility (Trail) [EB/OL].http://www.gov.cn/zhengce/zhengceku/2020-02/11/content5477301.htm

[8] West China Hospital, Sichuan University. Medical panel forCOVID-19 pneumonia of Sichuan Province. Emergency Prevention Guide for COVid-19 Pneumonia medical Institution [M]. Chengdu Sichuan Science and Technology Press, 2020.

[9] State Council of the People's Republic of China Notice on Conducting Proper and Precise Prevention and Control of COVID9EpidemicAccordingtoLaw.[eb/ol].http://www.nhcgov.cn/jkj/s3577/202002/69b3fdcbb61f-499ba50a25cdfl d5374e.shtml

[10] Ly Zhanxiu, Zhou Xianzhi, et al. Management of Modern Infectious Disease Hospital Beijing: People's Military Medical Press. 2010.

[11] Huang Gang, Lou Tianzheng, et al. Hand book of COVID-19Prevention and Treatment for Hospital at Community Level [M]. Hangzhou: Zhejiang University Press.

[12] National Health Commission of the People's Republic of China Dietary and Nutritional Guide for COVID-19 Prevention and Treatment [EB/OL].http://www.nhc.gov.cn/xcs/yqfk dt202002/a69fd36d54514c5a9a34456l88cbc428.shtml

[13] Hu Bijie, Liu Ronghui, et al. Diagram for SIFIC Hospital Infection Prevention and Control [M]. Shanghai: Shanghai Science and Technology Press, 2015.

[14] National Health Commission of the People's Republic of China Intervention

Guide for Emergency Psychological Crisis Caused by COVID-19 Epidemic [EB/OL] .http://www.nhc.gov.cn/j/s3577202001/6adc08b966594253b2b-791be5c3b9467.shtml

[15] Hubei Province Health Committee, Hubei Provincial Department of Education, Hubei Provincial Department of Finance, Hubei Resources and Social Security Department of Hubei Province. Measures on strengthening care and incentives for healthcare workers on frontline of COVId-19 prevention and control [EB/OL]. http://www.hubeigov.cn//zfwj/ezbf/202002/t202002182103386.shtml

Acknowledgements

Jack Ma Foundation

Alibaba Foundation

The Eighth Hospital of Wuhan

Wuhan Hanyang Hospital

Huanggang Central Hospital

Panlongcheng Branch of Huangpi District People's Hospital

The Second People's Hospital of Luotian County

People's Hospital of Jianli County

Suizhou Central Hospital